Medical Professionalism
in the New Information Age

Medical Professionalism in the New Information Age

Edited by
David J. Rothman and David Blumenthal

Rutgers University Press

New Brunswick, New Jersey, and London

Library of Congress Cataloging-in-Publication Data

Medical professionalism in the new information age / edited by David J. Rothman and David Blumenthal.

     p. ; cm. — (Critical issues in health and medicine)

  Includes bibliographical references and index.

  ISBN 978–0–8135–4807–4 (hardcover : alk. paper) — ISBN 978–0–8135–4808–1 (pbk. : alk. paper)

   1. Medical informatics.   2. Medical policy.   3. Medicine—Practice.   I. Rothman, David J.   II. Blumenthal, David, 1948–   III. Series: Critical issues in health and medicine.

  [DNLM: 1. Medical Informatics—trends—United States.   2. Professional Practice—trends—United States. W 26.5 M4899 2010]

  R858.M46   2010

  610.285—dc22

                              2009048327

A British Cataloging-in-Publication record for this book is available from the British Library.

Visit our Web site: http://rutgerspress.rutgers.edu

Manufactured in the United States of America

Contents

Acknowledgments

This project would not have come to fruition without the intellectual and administrative contributions of David Mechanic and Lynn Rogut in their capacities as director and deputy director of Rutgers State University Institute for Health, Health Care Policy and Aging Research. Working with the staff at Rutgers University Press was a delight; we would like to give particular thanks to Doreen Valentine, Caroline Hannaway, and Marilyn Campbell. Overseeing the project for us was Frederica Stahl, Research Associate at the Center of Medicine as a Profession. Her diligence, persistence, and skill made the final project all the more compelling.

Abbreviations

AAPC	American Academy of Professional Coders
ACOG	American College of Obstetricians and Gynecologists
AFEHCT	Association for Electronic Healthcare Transactions
AHA	American Hospital Association
AHIMA	American Health Information Management Association
AHRQ	Agency for Healthcare Research and Quality
AMA	American Medical Association
AMDIS	Association of Medical Directors of Information Systems
AMIA	American Medical Informatics Association
ART	Assisted Reproductive Technologies
BLS	Bureau of Labor Statistics
CAHIIM	Commission on Accreditation for Health Informatics and Information Management Education
CCHIT	Certifying Commission for Health Information Technology
CDC	Centers for Disease Control and Prevention
CHIM	Center for Healthcare Information Management
CHIME	College of Healthcare Information Management Executives
CMS	Center for Medicare and Medicaid Services
CMSS	Council of Medical Specialty Societies
CPHIMS	Certified Professional in Healthcare Information and Management Systems
CR	Consumers' Research
CU	Consumers Union
DHHS	Department of Health and Human Services
EDI	Electronic data exchange
EFM	Electronic fetal monitoring
HER	Electronic health record
ERISA	Employee Retirement Income Security Act
ESRD	End stage renal disease
FDA	Food and Drug Administration
FOIA	Freedom of Information Act
HCAHPS	Health Consumer Assessment of Health Care Providers and Systems
HCFA	Health Care Finance Administration
HEDIS	Healthcare Effectiveness Data and Information Set
HIET	Health information exchange technologies

Introduction

As we write this introduction, President Barack Obama has signed the American Recovery and Reinvestment Act of 2009 into law. This nearly $800 billion effort to shore up the foundering U.S. economy will have diverse and unpredictable effects, but one certain consequence is the wiring of our health care system. Between $14 and $27 billion of the $800 billion will go toward supporting—financially, logistically, technically—the acquisition and use of electronic health records (EHRs) by the nation's health care providers, including physicians and hospitals. An investment in EHRs on this scale was inconceivable before November 4, 2008, and before the collapse of the U.S. economy. Now there seems to be no turning back.

President Obama, his aides, and legislators of both political parties are hoping that the spread of EHRs will yield huge dividends in terms of the quality and efficiency of our health care system. That is a wish that all Americans likely share. But at the same time, a social investment of this size and novelty inevitably raises questions about unanticipated consequences, both positive and negative. In this volume, we explore one such possible effect: the implications of health information technology (HIT)—of which EHRs are just one example—for the profession of medicine, and in particular, for the professionalism of physicians.

At first glance, this may seem an odd direction in which to take discussions of HIT. Most of the literature in the field tilts toward economic, clinical and technical analysis: how to design the best electronic records; how to protect patient privacy and data security; and how to ensure that EHRs positively affect quality and reduce costs. We are asking a different but equally important set of questions: how will EHRs or other digital innovations fundamentally change the nature of medical practice, the professionalism of physicians, their relationships with patients, and their status in society? The practice of medicine has survived centuries of technological change, bending new technologies to its own and its patients' purposes and emerging more secure, powerful, and effective as a profession. Is health information technology just another in a long line of such advances, or will it create genuinely novel challenges and opportunities?

Each of the authors of the chapters that follow is convinced that this new technology will test the profession in unusual ways. To understand why, we need to focus attention on the foundations of physicians' role and status in society. These foundations rest preeminently on a unique competence—namely, the ability to master and marshal scientific information and technical skill for the purpose of caring and healing. This unique competence creates the profession's value and authority, and also forms the rationale for other professional obligations: to self-regulate and to embrace a moral and ethical code of conduct. Self-regulation is necessary because no group outside the profession is fully competent to judge the competence and skill of physicians. Embracing a moral and ethical code is necessary because the asymmetry of information between physicians and patients makes the latter vulnerable to exploitation by the former. Only if the profession conforms to ethical standards can patients be assured that they can trust their physicians, and trust is essential to effective care.

HIT, however, may conceivably weaken the traditional pillars of professional medical authority and the rationale for professionalism. The increased availability of health information online—including a growing trend to provide patients access to their own electronic health records and to enable them to develop personal health records that they control—could reduce the informational advantage that physicians traditionally have had over patients. By democratizing access to information, HIT may reduce or eliminate the asymmetries of information that have justified professional codes of conduct and that have also motivated patients to seek out physicians and to reimburse them for their services. Non-physician providers may also acquire increased authority in this environment, as they use computer prompts and guidance to provide advice. Consumers may find that instead of calling their physician and awaiting a response, they prefer to log on to an online help center that can immediately answer many of their specific questions. Decision-support software provided by companies like Google and Microsoft may help patients interpret health information without the guiding hand of a physician—especially a physician who is all too often rushed, harried, and inaccessible.

05-11-16 11:05AM

The item below is now available for pickup at designated location.

West Bloomfield Twp PL
zv350 West Bloomfield Pub Lib MAIN

Baker - Allen Park
CALL NO: R858 .M46 2010
AUTHOR:
Medical professionalism in the new
BARCODE: 33504005807880
REC NO: i345192874
PICKUP AT: Main Library Lobby

STEPHEN BERTMAN
Main

248-661-5948

7:1

Thus, HIT may be a destabilizing and disruptive technology in ways that few previous technological advances have been. It may fundamentally alter traditional relationships between physicians and patients, physicians and other providers of health care services, and physicians and the institutions with and for which they work. Whether these changes will actually occur, and whether they will be positive or negative, is very difficult to predict—only by thinking hard about them can we even posit the questions that could guide our consideration in going forward. And that, first and foremost, is the task that this volume sets for itself: thinking hard about the relationships among health information technology, the medical profession, and the larger society in a time of accelerating change.

To this end, the chapters in this volume explore subjects ranging from HIT's likely impact on the quality of care to consumer use and misuse of Web-based medical information and on to the need to reconsider the principles of medical liability. No one doubts the awesome power of HIT, but whether it will enhance or undermine medical professionalism and optimal medical care remains to be seen.

The project had its origins in 2004 at the annual meeting of the Robert Wood Johnson Health Policy Investigators. It grew out of casual conversations, not a specific program agenda, the happy result of bringing together diverse groups of health policy analysts. The informal discussions begun at one meeting became a more formal session at another, and then at another. Before long, the Robert Wood Johnson Policy Foundation (through the efforts of David Mechanic and Lynn Rogut) and the Institute on Medicine as a Profession became the joint sponsors of this project. Courtesy of this endeavor, the authors learned a great deal about the special problems posed by HIT, and our hope is that readers of this book will as well. One caveat, however, must be added: the chapters are better at raising intriguing questions rather than offering confident predictions.

The opening chapter by David Blumenthal provides an overview of the current state of HIT, first outlining its implications for patients' access to their own information, patients' access to physician-generated information (patient charts), and billing information. Blumenthal then focuses on the implications of HIT for the patient-physician relationship, explaining why physicians are at once excited by and in dread of the technology. In his view, accessible personal health records, transferable electronic health records, and the rapid and ever-present flow of health information on the Internet may well undermine physicians' traditional claim to unique knowledge and technical competence. But in the end, he is optimistic about the likely impact of HIT on medical professionalism. As information technology provides patients with plausible diagnosis and treatment options, medical practice will change. Physicians will come to recognize and appreciate their new role as guides, information management experts, not as the first and last word as decision makers.

The next two chapters focus attention on the impact of HIT on the organization and oversight of medical care. Mark Hall and Kristin Madison see significant opportunities for improvement. They point out that physicians will come under a professional obligation to facilitate data collection and measurement efforts that will enhance medical regulation by external forces and improve the quality of medical guidelines. HIT will promote transparency, with significant benefits for the delivery of care. Physicians will have little choice but to become deeply involved in the development of regulatory and measurement tools, such as provider report cards and pay-for-performance programs—otherwise they will lose the power to shape their own professional identity and practices. Hall and Madison encourage physicians to take up this charge, explaining that the new regulatory apparatus can strengthen three fundamental principles of medical professionalism: the primacy of patient welfare, respect for patient autonomy, and a commitment to promote social justice.

Nancy Tomes has a more skeptical position on HIT's ability to ensure quality care. She places the technology in a broad historical context, emphasizing, in particular, the forty-year-old consumer movement and its relationship to health care. She moves from consumer guides like Zagat to print and electronic media like *U.S. News and World Report* to advocacy organizations and health system analysts like *Public Citizen* and the *Dartmouth Atlas* to convey a sense of how varied and extensive the data collection and promulgation enterprise already is. But Tomes takes issue with the common perception that publicly accessible information is a prescription to remedy the ailing health care system. She notes that many interventions, including ratings of doctors and hospitals, often have unintended consequences—patients make some use of the information, but health care marketers and advertisers make even greater use. Appreciating the extraordinary advantages that come from an electronic system for compiling and analyzing data, Tomes still questions whether "information fixes" are adequate to address the problems consumers confront with so many stakeholders and such complex rules. Indeed, she wonders whether by undermining the profession's self-regulation and monopoly on valued knowledge, HIT will end up strengthening the very market forces that professionalism was supposed to overcome.

The following two chapters examine the likely impact of HIT on professional responsibility and behavior from the vantage point of law as well as medicine. Sara Rosenbaum and Michael Painter address how new forms of information distribution are likely to affect legal liability cases. Invoking the case of the *T. J. Hooper*, where tugboat owners were found negligent in an accident for not having radio communications technology on board, they argue that IT may well soon become the equivalent of the radio, not just encouraging but compelling physicians to adopt HIT. Given the value and ease of the adoption, physicians who resist may find themselves liable for not having an IT system. Rosenbaum and Painter go on to suggest that HIT may also create new expectations about the quality of health information and transparency. Physicians will be required to submit the clinical decisions they have made (prescriptions, diagnostic tests, etc.) to their groups and their patients, both to ensure the quality of their care and to inform not only their patients, but all patients—that is, the society at large. Indeed, if under the umbrella of HIT, medicine becomes a public rather than only a patient-centered activity, a no-fault compensation system might replace the traditional medical tort system for liability.

Marc Rodwin's chapter also explores how data collected through HIT might be used to enhance medical decision making through the creation of a database on outcomes, injuries, and side effects. Patient data, he too insists, should be made to serve the public good. However, the only way to accomplish this end is through public, not private, ownership of patient data, an issue that the law has not yet fully addressed. At the moment, innovation is stifled by private property rights which now cover the collection of health care data. Rodwin believes that both policy makers and medical professionals should join forces to change this paradigm so as to create more manageable and uniform datasets. Although Rodwin recognizes that effective federal regulation would go a long way to accomplishing this goal, he is very much aware that private data-mining companies are aligned against it, and not for the first or last time, these companies may win out. Nevertheless, there are useful models already to be found, including the data collected by the Veterans Health Administration, Geisinger Health System, and Kaiser Permanente. Because the public good would be so well served by this change, he is hopeful that the commons will triumph over private interests.

The book moves next to two in-depth case studies of how HIT is already affecting doctor-patient relationships and medical professionalism. In both instances, patients eagerly employ the technology, but they do so in ways that may contravene both physicians' interests and social welfare.

Sheila M. Rothman, Natassia M. Rozario, and David J. Rothman examine how patients with end stage renal disease who are searching for a kidney for transplantation marshal HIT to their own advantage. Web sites, such as matchingdonors.org, allow them to enter an ostensibly non-commercial space to meet their need. On this site, and others as well, patients post personal information, unverified, to attract potential living donors; by the same token, would-be donors may present themselves as altruistic but, in fact, may be looking for financial or other rewards. The Internet-based search for a kidney assumes many of the characteristics of the search for a date or a child to adopt—exaggeration and duplicity can become the coin of the realm. Yet, at the same time, the use of the Internet has broadened the scope of possibilities for a patient in search of an organ. It allows for a dramatic expansion of social networks, reaching well beyond immediate family and community. More, and this should not be taken lightly, would-be recipients of an organ are far more comfortable in reaching out to strangers for a donation than putting a burden on relatives and friends who are part of their intimate circle.

All the while, Web-based exchanges between strangers present novel challenges to transplant teams and organizations, which they are having difficulty meeting. How closely should they examine the circumstances behind the donation transaction? Can they simply accept the organ and run the risk of circumventing fundamental ethical and legal principles? It appears that transplant teams and organizations are grappling with the implications of patient-donor use of the Internet for maintaining the key principles of medical professionalism.

The second case study by Eugene Declercq explores HIT in the context of maternity practices. Informative maternal health Web sites have significantly influenced women's preferences on the childbirth experience; one in six new mothers turns to the Internet as the primary information source for pregnancy and birth. Declercq asks how this practice affects physician authority and behavior. On the one hand, the change in the sources of information may well be encouraging obstetricians, who once managed a very consumer-focused and time-consuming relationship with their patients, to practice in groups, sharing patients among a number of professionals. On the other, historically the profession responded to external challenges, such as the revival of midwifery and at-home birth, by either co-opting the movements or by establishing a language and theory of pregnancy that reasserted the need for professional oversight. As the information available to mothers expands, it is not at all certain, Declercq concludes, that the profession will be able to circumvent the effects of this newest technology.

In the book's closing chapter, Mark C. Suchman and Matthew Dimick look to the future. They are persuaded that HIT is creating a health-information profession which is distinct from medicine. They summarize the attributes of a profession and then fit HIT practitioners to the model. On the basis of the number of people involved, their collective self-awareness, the journals they publish, the conferences they run, and the organizations that support them, it is apparent that HIT is a profession in the making. Suchman and Dimick go on to note that this new cadre stands between physicians and clinical care personnel (devoted to improving patient outcomes), and hospital and insurance company managers (promoting network order and security and giving precedence to group and system needs). Physicians, for example, may find keeping a "shadow chart" in their desk harmless and convenient; to information technology professionals, it represents a basic threat to the integrity of the data system. Where HIT personnel will eventually fit remains uncertain, but anyone concerned with professionalism will have to chart their location.

Taken together, the chapters in this book identify the crucial transformations that health information technology may well bring. The changes, by necessity, will destabilize the status quo, with foreseen and unforeseen consequences. If the profession rises to the challenge, HIT has the potential to promote the delivery of higher quality, evidence-based, and better regulated medicine. The alternative is to have physicians stand apart from and resist the march of technology, an unacceptable outcome medically, legally, and socially. Physicians will have to adapt information technology to their practices, recognizing that they as well as their patients and the larger society will benefit from a technologically integrated and sophisticated medical system. Put most succinctly, the use of HIT has to become another marker of medical professionalism.

Expecting the Unexpected

Health Information Technology
and Medical Professionalism

The medical profession—in various manifestations—has survived and thrived since the beginning of recorded history. It now sits astride an industry that accounts for 8 to 16 percent of the gross domestic product of most developed countries, and its scientific armamentarium grows constantly, as does its command of societal resources. Over time, it has sought out and absorbed a vast array of technologies to treat illness, from bloodletting leeches to proton beam therapy.[1]

Now the medical profession confronts still another innovation in the long list of technological opportunities: health information technology (HIT). Based on the profession's past success in managing new technology, HIT ought to produce bored yawns from physicians contemplating its adoption in their profession, but instead, it is provoking something quite different: a mixture of excitement and dread. Those who welcome HIT and those who fear it seem to have one thing in common: both camps view it as potentially transformational for the health care system. Indeed, the prospect of a wired health care world has become a kind of Rorschach test, distinguishing physician optimists from physician pessimists. Optimists anticipate an idealized world of health care perfection in which their work becomes almost miraculously efficient and effective. Pessimists foresee an endless struggle in their daily work in which their patients drop sheaves of misleading Internet print-outs on their desks, bureaucrats torture them with irrelevant, beeping reminders and monitor their every move, and software glitches paralyze them as their waiting rooms seethe with angry patients.

Finding clarity amidst these contending fantasies is a difficult task, but an important one. The potential impact of HIT on physicians and their professional identity is important to understand for many reasons, not the least of which is that patients today continue to view their relationships with physicians as vital to their health and well-being. Thus, any technology that has the potential fundamentally to alter those relationships is of more than passing interest. Our track record of predicting the effects of much more constrained and limited technologies on medicine and health care has not been spectacular, so we should enter any exercise in conjecture regarding HIT with humility: best to expect the unexpected. Nevertheless, we may gain some modest insight into the future impact of HIT on the medical profession by addressing the following questions:

What is health information technology?

What is its current status within the U.S. health care system?

What is the potential range of effects that HIT will have on physicians, health systems, and patients?

What impact will these effects have on the medical profession and the relationships of physicians with patients?

One assumption underlies much of the discussion here: human nature changes much more slowly than technology, and one enduring aspect of human nature is the desire for a soothing hand and dependable expert advice during times of illness and anxiety. Men and women want care from other men and women—and not from robotic imitations thereof—when they are sick. If doctors respond appropriately, these human instincts give physicians an enormous opportunity to use HIT to define and support a new, more powerful professional identity and more dynamic, more effective relationships with patients.

What Is HIT?

Health information technology consists of a vast and rapidly changing array of electronic methods for collecting, storing, manipulating, and deploying the information that supports the functioning of our health care system. This chapter will concern itself with technologies for managing patient-specific clinical information, but there are many other applications of HIT: billing systems, computer applications used in advanced imaging, bar coding, supply chain management, and so on. Each of these applications can affect the cost and quality of care. But for the role and status of doctors and the medical profession, the technologies that affect physicians' clinical decisions and their interactions with patients are the most salient.

These technologies fall into three general categories: the electronic health record (EHR), the personal health record (PHR), and health information exchange technologies (HIET) that enable data to pass between and among EHRs and PHRs.

Electronic health records are what most people think of first when HIT comes to mind. EHRs are systems that support physicians in the care of individual patients. According to the Institute of Medicine, eight capabilities or functionalities define an EHR. These include the ability to collect patient demographic data, to store and display clinical information (such as medications, symptom lists, diagnoses, laboratory results, and so on), to enter orders (electronic prescriptions for tests and treatments), to provide support for decisions on treatment (such as drug interactions and access to guidelines), to interact with other EHRs (through HIET systems), to communicate with patients (via electronic mail), to generate billing data and other administrative services, and to support key public health functions (such as reporting of infectious diseases). Currently, many commercial vendors provide EHR systems, and the federal government is creating a process for certifying EHRs to ensure that they have certain basic, essential features.

Personal health records are less defined and refined than EHRs, though their potential to transform the health care system and to affect the medical profession is as profound. PHRs currently come in three forms. The first is sometimes called the personally controlled health record (PCHR). The PCHR is what comes to mind for many people when they think of a PHR. The PCHR enables patients to keep and control all their own health care data. They could maintain these data on a CD, a hard drive, a flash drive, or a secure Web site constructed for this purpose. Both Microsoft and Google have launched applications intended to offer consumers the means to do precisely this. One of the PCHR's major attractions is that it ensures that patients can make available their health information to whomever they want, whenever they want. The PCHR could radically change the balance of power between physicians and patients by giving the latter control over information previously assembled and dispensed by doctors and by enabling patients to make better use of nonmedical sources of advice, diagnosis, and treatment.

A second and more commonly available version of the PHR enables patients to gain access to some or all of the data about them maintained by doctors and health care organizations. Also known as a patient portal or gateway, it leaves control of the patient's information in the provider's hands, but employs electronic technology to share that data with patients. A number of health care systems maintain patient portals, including Kaiser Permanente,

Table 1.1   Basic EHR Functions Necessary to Promote Patient Safety, As Defined by the Institute of Medicine

Core Functionalities	Key Elements
Health Information and Data: patient information needed to make sound clinical decisions	Medical and nursing diagnoses, medication lists, allergies, demographics, clinical narratives, and test results
Results Management: ability to manage results of all types electronically	Computerized laboratory test results and radiology procedure result reports, automated display of previous and current test results
Order Entry Management: entry of medication and other care orders, as well as ancillary services, directly into a computer	Computerized physician order entry (CPOE); patient laboratory, microbiology, pathology, radiology orders; electronic prescribing of medication orders; nursing orders; ancillary service and consult referrals
Decision Support: computer reminders and prompts to improve prevention, diagnosis, and management of patient disease	Screening for correct drug selection, dosing, and interactions of chosen drugs with other medications; preventive health reminders for vaccinations, breast cancer screening, colorectal screening, and cardiovascular risk detection; clinical guidelines and pathways for patient treatment; management of chronic diseases
Electronic Communication and Connectivity: online communication between the health care team, other care partners, and patients	Electronic communication tools—including integrated health records, e-mail, and Web messaging—for use among health care team members, between physicians, laboratories, radiology and pharmacies, and with patients; telemedicine or electronic communications between providers and patients who reside in remote areas; home telemonitoring for the elderly or others with chronic diseases
Patient Support: education and self-testing	Computer-based patient education; home telemonitoring for patients with chronic diseases
Administrative Processes: electronic scheduling systems and billing and claims management	Electronic scheduling systems for hospital admissions, inpatient and outpatient procedures, and visits; validation of insurance eligibility, claim authorization, and prior approvals; identification of patients eligible for clinical trials
Reporting and Population Health Management: clinical data collection to meet public, private, and institutional requirements	Clinical data represented with standardized terminology and in a machine-readable format to meet federal, state, local, and public health reporting requirements; also to meet organizational reporting requirements for key quality indicators

Source: Institute of Medicine, *Key Capabilities of an Electronic Health Record System* (Washington, DC: National Academies Press, 2003).

the Veterans Health Administration, Vanderbilt Medical Center in Nashville, the Beth Israel Deaconess Medical Center in Boston, and the Palo Alto Medical Group in the San Francisco Bay Area.

The third type of PHR has been developed by insurance companies and health plans. These technologies give clients of these organizations access to information gleaned from billing data. Such information might include lists of problems, medications, the status of various preventive and screening tests, and appraisals of the quality and cost of care patients have received to the extent that quality and cost can be assessed from claims and other information accessible to health plans. Obviously, this third type of PHR is much less robust than the first two, since it generally lacks the detailed clinical records that are contained in the PCHR or are accessible through patient portals. However, insurance companies increasingly see themselves as information management companies, not just as underwriters or claims processors, and they are seeking to sell information services to clients. Therefore, with their huge resources, these firms can be expected to promote their versions of PHRs widely.

The third general type of HIT referred to above, health information exchange technology, is the most abstract of the three, and largely functions in the background. However, it is important for realizing the potential of EHRs and PHRs. HIET enables EHRs maintained by different organizations and doctors to communicate, usually over the Web, so that all of a patient's data, regardless of when and where they were collected, can be combined in one place. HIET also enables EHRs and PHRs to connect, which is crucial if PHRs are to stay up to date, and vice versa.

The Current Status of HIT

HIT is not yet widely available in the United States. As of early 2008, 13 percent of U.S. physicians had EHRs with the basic functionalities that define this technology.[2] Another 4 percent had advanced EHRs that might be called fully functional. The figure for hospitals is closer to 10 percent.[3] PHRs are vanishingly rare—fewer than 5 percent of the U.S. population has access to these at the current time, and the most common form is the patient portal or the insurance company-based version of a PHR. HIET is not common either. Somewhere between 100 and 200 communities are exploring the creation of systems for health information exchange, but only a handful have created functioning networks.[4]

The United States lags far behind many European nations in its adoption of HIT, though comparative data suffer from inconsistent definitions of particular technologies and from uncertainty about the validity of information in particular

Table 1.2   **Percentage of General Practitioners with Office Computers**

Australia	98%	Netherlands	97%
Austria	99%	New Zealand	100%
Denmark	99%	Norway	100%
England	99%	Scotland	95%
Germany	90%	Sweden	97%

Source: Denis Protti, G. Wright, S. Treweek, and I. Johansen, "Primary Care Computing in England and Scotland: A Comparison with Denmark," *Inform Primary Care* 14 (2006): 93–99.

countries. In most developed nations, primary care physicians—usually general practitioners—are much more likely to have EHRs than in the United States.[5]

This difference between the United States and other nations reflects a variety of factors, but it seems clear that government leadership has played an important role in most nations where most primary care physicians use EHRs. With the enactment of the Health Information Technology for Clinical and Economic Health Act (HITECH) of 2009, part of the so-called "Recovery Act" enacted in February 2009, the U.S. federal government has for the first time assumed that leadership responsibility.

A government role is essential because of considerable obstacles to private adoption of HIT. Individual physicians and small groups have been reluctant to lay out the monies required to implement EHRs, which can total $15,000 to $50,000 per physician. There has been little patient demand for PHRs, so the field has been left to crusading health care organizations that are committed to providing patients access to their records out of a sense that this is the right thing to do, or will enhance their market share in the future. Indeed, HIET has many of the aspects of a public good. Even organizations that see benefits to equipping their own physicians with EHRs are likely to see little gain in connecting to wider networks. After all, sharing patient data just makes it easier for their patients to use other providers.

HITECH addresses a number of the barriers to HIT adoption in the U.S., and will undoubtedly speed its spread. The question, therefore, is what an HIT-enabled future will have in store for the medical profession.

The Likely Effects of HIT

How might physicians prepare themselves now for a future in which HIT is ubiquitous and far more powerful than it currently is? This is not wholly an academic exercise. Students currently entering medical school will reach the peak of their professional skill and productivity in twenty-five years, and will likely remain in practice for more than forty. Therefore, they will be living the future that this author is currently trying to anticipate. Since the nature and effects of HIT will vary with the type and location of care, this chapter focuses for simplicity on primary care practice to illustrate the changes that HIT will enable and catalyze.

First, the workplaces of primary care providers (with the possible exception of nursing homes, which have been especially slow to adopt HIT) will be paperless. Everything providers know about patients, and everything they do with and for them, will be mediated by software. The computer will be as omnipresent and important as the stethoscope.

Second, patients' records will be accessible at all times to providers in secure digital locations approved by the patient and to whomever else the patient grants access. This will certainly be true within countries and likely internationally as well. The era of the lost or inaccessible chart will be over.

Third, patients' interactions with care providers and the work flow of provider offices and organizations will change dramatically. Patients will connect with care providers online and many routine issues will be handled without direct provider-patient contact. These will include such matters as obtaining prescription renewals, arranging for referrals and appointments, managing third-party authorizations, and tracking paperwork, and so on. Prior to office visits, many patients will receive e-mail notification to go to provider Web sites to fill out questionnaires covering such matters as their chief complaint, symptoms, and current medications, and to confirm important elements of past medical history and changes in medical condition since their last visit to the provider. For patients who wish to perform these tasks orally, voice recognition software will take the necessary information and then other software will extract the relevant data from the verbal input. Artificial intelligence will use new and existing patient data to pose additional questions to patients that will help to confirm or refute hypotheses about patients' diagnoses. For many routine problems, the online logic will present the patient with a diagnosis and treatment plan (cold/Tylenol; itching between toes/anti-fungal cream), and the patient will be allowed to choose whether to follow the recommendations or to seek a face-to-face appointment. A third option might be an e-mail, a phone call, or a video conference with a nurse practitioner or with a physician to resolve uncertainties. For more complicated or worrisome problems, such as chest pain or severe shortness of breath, a few key questions will determine whether the patient should be advised to visit their nearest emergency department.

When patients need to be seen in a physician's office in order to make an accurate diagnosis and to plan or provide therapy—or when patients simply choose a personal visit—they will arrive with a large amount of work having been accomplished through the online screening process. This will greatly increase the efficiency and quality of office practice. Of course, physicians will have the option to consider other hypotheses, collect additional data, and change the specified plans suggested prior to the visit. But in many cases, they will just certify what the patient's e-consultation advised. For chronically ill patients, the information available to the patient and providers will include the results of home monitoring of key physiological parameters: weight for congestive heart failure patients, blood pressure for hypertensives, blood sugars for diabetics, clotting parameters for patients on blood thinners. Telemonitoring these parameters will enable the patient and his or her medical team to improve control over chronic illness—or at least, will provide that patient with much more intelligent and continuous advice between office visits. In many cases, patients, assisted by software that monitors their personal data, will be able to change medications by themselves, following guidelines available online or agreed to in advance with their health care providers.

Fourth, for patients who wish to be full partners in their care, the information available to them will be vast. They will have access to all of their personal health information online, and that information will be interpreted for them using decision support provided by their commercial PHR vendor. In return for this service, patients will allow the vendor to display "pop-up" advertisements targeted to their personal health and search profiles. Some patients may prefer to pay a fee for their PHR service, and thereby avoid the annoyance and intrusiveness of advertising. Others may subscribe to advertisement-free PHRs maintained by their health care organizations. PHR vendors will offer their paying customers a menu of specialized services. These may include health advisories that reflect a patient's demographic or personal health information (a reminder that it is time for a colonoscopy or a flu shot, for example), quality and cost ratings of local physicians and hospitals (the patient's local hospital has an excellent carotid endarterectomy service; for bypass, try going elsewhere), and price lists for pharmaceuticals at local pharmacies. Patients will have a variety of options for managing their personal health information: they may grant blanket access to all care providers within a designated organization or provide access on a case-by-case basis, for example, to a specialist to whom they are referred. PHR vendors will make lucrative deals with high profile health care organizations with national brands—Mayo, Hopkins, M. D. Anderson—to provide endorsements for their sites and services. These organizations will also receive preferred treatment on the Web site to encourage referrals to these facilities.

Fifth, the nature of face-to-face physician-patient contacts will be significantly modified by HIT. Aside from the usual benefits of HIT—ready availability of clinical data from any source, decision support, easily printable patient education material—electronic technologies will be a constant, though hopefully unobtrusive, presence in the physician-patient interaction. Much of the process of data retrieval and input may be voice-activated, and digital image records of patient encounters will also be important sources of ongoing data and quality control (ultrasound records, actual audio recordings of patient descriptions of symptoms). At the same time, physicians will receive a constant stream of advice—if they choose to use it—concerning how to process and respond to information about the patients they are seeing. How to manage these resources will come to be a signature aspect of primary care physicians' practice style and a critical influence on the quality of care they provide. Health care organizations may distinguish themselves in part by the manner in which they support and train their physicians and other health professionals to use computerized decision support and the many online resources that are available for use in patient care.

Sixth, as important as patient-physician interaction will be the effect of HIT on communication among care providers. At the simplest level, HIT will enable all providers involved in patients' care to have access to colleagues' notes and actions, both within and across health care organizations and communities. At a more sophisticated level, new software may facilitate group management of patients that is more productive and efficient than is currently possible. Consider this scenario: A home monitoring device detects deterioration in a patient's blood pressure control. Decision support suggests that the patient increase or change a medication, but after a week on the new regimen, no benefit results. The decision support then directs a series of pertinent questions and prompts simultaneously each member of the patient's care team to respond with an analysis or recommendation. The patient's nurse practitioner may be prompted to contact the patient about dietary salt consumption, any change in his or her exercise routine or weight gain. The physician will receive an advisory noting that the patient is already on three medicines for anti-hypertensive control, and that should the nurse not find a readily preventable cause of deterioration, the physician should consider treatable medical causes of hypertension, such as renal artery stenosis or bilateral adrenal hyperplasia. The physician will receive a reminder if the nurse has tried and failed to control the patient's blood pressure, and orders for the necessary tests to check for treatable medical causes of hypertension will be entered automatically. The physician can choose to sign the orders or not, can schedule a patient visit, or both. The nurse will be notified of the physician's decision by incoming e-mail. In this way, HIT will deploy health care teams in a coordinated assault on patients' health care problems.

Implications for Professionalism

In projecting the possible effects of health information technology on the nature of medical care, we are limited only by our imaginations, and by the defiant tendency of humans and human systems to act in totally unexpected ways. Sometimes, the logical and efficient runs counter to the way humans *actually* think and feel (as opposed to the way system engineers believe people *should* think and feel) and promising ideas flounder. For example, it is quite possible that current efforts to use HIT to make patients "full partners" in managing their own illnesses will stall in the face of many patients' deep-seated desire to be cared for by other human beings (rather than by themselves), and to the enormous deficits in health care literacy that affect so many Americans. When large segments of the population do not understand what "percent" means, relying on individuals to make good decisions in response to self-generated health care data may be a challenge.

Nevertheless, HIT is coming, and it will cause significant change. The question here is: what does this mean for the medical profession generally, and for professionalism in particular? It is necessary first to dispel one myth. HIT will not cause physicians to become obsolete, replaced perhaps by robotically pleasant online "communications specialists" whose real job is just to direct patients to the right Web site. For at least the next thirty years or so, flesh and blood physicians will continue to be critical participants in the health care system. They will continue to see patients, and patients will continue to rely on them in times of need.

A few examples are sufficient to make this point. For the foreseeable future, highly trained health professionals will be needed for both diagnostic and therapeutic tasks: to feel patients' bellies to assess exactly where and how intense the pain is; to see whether a sore joint is swollen, red, and tender (indicating infection or arthritis) or whether it is unstable (indicating traumatic injury); to see whether a patient has lost sensation in a leg afflicted by sciatica; to weave a catheter through the artery in the leg up into the heart and to decide, in real time, whether and where to place a stent in a coronary artery; and to remove a colonic polyp via colonoscopy. All these tasks require the physician's touch and are as yet beyond the capacity of automated systems to perform.

However, the fact that physicians will remain important to medicine is no guarantee of complacency for the profession. To see where and how the profession and professionalism will change, it is helpful to review the core attributes that undergird professional status in medicine. These attributes are threefold:

> Physicians should maintain a unique technical competence that adds value for patients.
>
> Physicians should undertake active self-regulation to assure conformance to professional norms.
>
> Physicians must be willing to put the interests of patients ahead of the professionals' own interests.

Professionalism is important to medicine because non-experts find it difficult to regulate and control groups with unique technical competence. Similarly, the ethical component of professional norms arises from the asymmetry of knowledge between patient and physician. The market's reliance on caveat emptor suffices where knowledge asymmetry is less profound.

The rise of HIT will affect all three pillars of professionalism, but first and most directly, health information technology will substantially alter physicians' traditional claims to unique technical competence. For reasons hinted at above, the challenge to these claims will arise first for the so-called "cognitive specialties" of medicine: those in which thinking rather than procedural interventions are the most important tasks. The reason, quite simply, is that HIT is further along in facilitating and mastering the work of information provision and processing than in mimicking the hand-eye coordination and spatial reasoning that are so critical to accomplishing invasive procedures. Thus, it will be generalist physicians—both primary care doctors and those specialists who manage the chronically ill—who will forge the way in grappling with and redefining the nature of professionalism in the age of new information technology.

It must be acknowledged, first, that the development of HIT will require (or enable) cognitively-based physicians to delegate many tasks that they previously held closely. The routine management of many uncomplicated chronic illnesses, and the treatment of many routine office complaints—these tasks will no longer require the services of professionals with eight years of formal schooling and at least three years of apprenticeship training. A nurse practitioner or a physician assistant—or even a college-trained medical technician—with computerized decision support (or without it in many cases) will be able to manage a substantial proportion of what used to take the time of generalists and even some specialists, such as diabetologists, pulmonologists, and rheumatologists. Of course, experts have long anticipated and advocated using non-physician health professionals to provide routine office care, and this development is already under way. HIT will merely accelerate and extend it.

More threatening for physicians (and other health professionals) will be the opportunity—and requirement—to delegate more decisions to patients themselves. As noted, not all patients will want to exercise, or be capable of exercising more control over the management of their acute and chronic conditions, but individuals who do may experience superior health outcomes at lower costs. Using home-monitoring devices and computerized algorithms, hypertensives, diabetics, and heart failure patients will be able to adjust their own medicines. For many patients with chronic illness, the locus of their care will move from the health care system to the kitchen table. In the process, they will become the real experts on their particular version of common conditions that are often quite variable in their effects on individual patients. The resulting speedy, personalized self-care will avoid physician visits, hospitalizations, prescription mishaps, and unnecessary diagnostic testing. But patient empowerment will also lead to reduced physician authority in the management of the bread-and-butter conditions of generalist physicians.

Physicians will also find themselves caring for an increasingly knowledgeable patient population in other ways. At almost every current physician-patient encounter, there is already a third presence in the room: the Web. A large proportion of patients with new complaints have already searched for hints as to what may be causing their back pain, perceived shortness of breath, headache, dizziness, swollen ankles, or rash. Those with questions about vaccinations or other preventive interventions will rarely arrive without an opinion about whether they should get that shot to prevent shingles or pneumonia, or that MRI for breast cancer. Sometimes, they will have entered their personal data into an online risk calculator that factors their age, family history, childhood exposure to radiation, known genotype, and previous test results into a prediction of the chance that they will get breast cancer, heart disease, or diabetes. In these cases, the first contact with medical professionals becomes equivalent to what used to be called a second opinion. The challenge for the physician only increases with the circumstances of modern medicine. Physicians no longer have the time to indulge in eliciting long histories. They could never in the past hope really to know patients and their symptoms as well as the patients themselves did, but now, patients will enjoy not only fuller knowledge of their own circumstances, but have much more decision support to help them process that knowledge into informed decisions.

These trends themselves are easier to discern than are their precise effects on physicians' claims to unique technical competence and thus to professional privileges and obligations. However, some tentative predictions seem plausible. First, over the next thirty years, "cognitive" physicians *will* continue to have a unique technical competence, and will continue to be important to patient care, but they will have to be smarter and more nimble in order to do so. Knowing the usual things, providing the usual services, will no longer suffice. Instead, physicians will assist their patients by providing consultations and advice that help patients refine complex decisions. Physicians will have to be smarter than their ever more knowledgeable patients. The race is on.

Second, it will be impossible for physicians to meet these challenges without help in several forms. The first will come from HIT itself: physicians should be—and will have to be—much more capable of using the Internet for health care purposes than their patients. After all, physicians spend all day worrying about and retrieving information about health care, while patients (except for the rare ones) will generally search episodically. Thus, physicians will assist their patients in part through mastering better than laypersons the exploding body of information on health and health care. This in turn will require that they be trained in using online information sources, and that they be supported with physician-specific, enhanced information systems that enable them to tap the full range of valid and useful Web-based information resources in real time.

An example of how not to be prepared for this challenge comes from my personal experience. A patient, who happens to be a professor of biology and who recently started a statin medication to lower his cholesterol, came into my office recently saying that he had read reports of research at Harvard Medical School showing how this medication caused a common side effect that he had experienced. He wanted to discuss the paper. I went online to find it, and could not, whereupon he informed me that he had located it easily by doing his own search. I was left looking like an amateur at health information retrieval—a completely accurate impression. In the future, this will not suffice. The ability to search quickly and accurately for health information will be a core element of technical competence for medical professionals.

Another source of support for physicians will come from health care organizations. Organizations will help physicians acquire, but even more important, learn to use the full potential of HIT. To be more knowledgeable than patients will require time for continuing training, and health care systems can help support the associated costs of this and arrange for necessary coverage. They can also help physicians scan the sources available for new knowledge and evaluate its importance for clinical care. To be smarter than their patients, physicians will need a little help from their friends.

Third, physicians will need to develop new forms of expertise that add value in an increasingly bewildering and rapidly changing health care environment. After all, the changes that physicians find so challenging will be even more challenging to patients who do not make a "profession" out of dealing with health care issues. Physicians will need skills as personal health navigators in ways that are sensitive to patients' needs, and much more relevant to the real challenges that patients face in managing their health and that of their families.

What does all this mean in practical terms? In the next thirty years, physicians may provide more assistance to their patients by helping them choose among alternative courses of treatment already known to the patient than by making a diagnosis and proposing those treatments. Physicians may add more value by checking the patient's logic than by supplying information, by identifying unlikely but important diagnoses that the patient's search may have discounted, or by changing the probabilities on the patients' own decision tree, based on physicians' greater experience with signs, symptoms, and laboratory tests. Physicians may also add enormous value by helping patients digest the increasingly complex and tortured data that will be available on the comparative performance of health care organizations and physicians, thus helping their patients make choices about how to navigate the health care system itself.

Another example of a patient encounter may be informative. I recently saw an executive in a consulting firm in my office with a complaint of pain in his right upper abdomen. This visit followed several days of e-mails in which he described his symptoms and asked for advice on what he should do. I advised him to be seen, but he at first demurred. When he eventually arrived, he told me he thought he had a gallbladder problem. Several siblings had had gallstones, his pain had started the morning after eating an unusually large fatty meal, and he was sore when he pushed on his stomach in the appropriate place. He had done a Web search, and everything seemed to fit. He wanted an abdominal ultrasound—the correct diagnostic test—to look for the gallstones he was sure he had.

But as I questioned him in more depth than was possible by e-mail, some things did not fit the diagnosis at all. One was that his pain increased when he breathed, and a second was that he was somewhat short of breath. Still a third symptom was that he had had a general feeling of muscle aching, as though he had the flu, the same day that his pain started. I realized that his formulation of the possible diagnoses was too limited, and added at least two others: pleuritis (an inflammation of the lining of the lung) and, more ominously, pulmonary embolus. The physical examination of the patient was normal except for some mild tenderness in the right upper area of his stomach on deep breathing—a finding that could, indeed, be consistent with gallbladder irritation. However, I felt that doing the ultrasound he wanted would not suffice, and added a chest

X-ray and a screening test for a pulmonary embolus to his work-up. In fact, he had a viral pleuritis—and no gallstones. The contribution of the medical professional here was to add to the patient's list of possible diagnoses, to sort them by likelihood, and to choose the additional tests necessary to exclude the other possibilities.

This portrait of the basis of technical competence—the fundamental foundation of medical professionalism—thirty years from now suggests several changes in the nature of the profession itself. First, physicians will have to be smarter than ever, and they will have to keep learning throughout their careers at an accelerating and demanding pace. Second, no matter how smart they are, they will need a lot of help from organized systems of care—whether real or virtual—that keep physicians supplied with the most advanced useable information on health care diagnoses and treatments. Third, they will have to be trained to adapt continually to a changing informational environment and a changing health care system. Fourth, the demand for traditional cognitive physician services will decline, and cognitive services themselves will become more specialized and harder to perform. We will likely have fewer, more specialized primary care physicians—think of them as ninja PCPs—who provide decision support for patients and supervise less-trained primary care providers, including nurses and physician assistants. The paradox of the future health system is that we will have much more primary care, and primary care will be more important than ever, but it will be supplied predominantly by patients and non-physicians, with backup from specialized primary care providers who are master diagnosticians and clinical decision makers, powered by health information and organizational supports.

As health information technology transforms the U.S. health care system, the profession will change, but professionalism will continue to be an essential ingredient in an ever-evolving health care system. Though HIT creates an apparent challenge to the unique status of the medical profession, it also provides the answer to that challenge.

Quality Regulation in the Information Age

Challenges for Medical Professionalism

Recent studies documenting continued deficiencies in health care quality have prompted a renewed commitment to developing regulatory tools well suited to addressing quality problems.[1] State governments in the United States have traditionally relied on the medical profession to exercise oversight over the quality of medical care by weeding out poor-quality providers through the licensure and professional discipline processes. More recently, however, improvements in information technology have facilitated alternative approaches to assessing and improving provider quality, such as provider report cards and pay-for-performance programs. While these tools have sometimes been criticized as inaccurate or ineffective, their use has been spreading.

Information technology-driven approaches to health care quality regulation have important implications for both individual physicians and the medical profession as a whole. For physicians, professional obligations to serve patient welfare, respect patient autonomy, and promote social justice impose a responsibility to improve quality tools and to ensure that patients benefit from them.[2]

For the medical profession, the information revolution raises doubts about the future of self-regulation. The widespread dissemination of information allows non-medical professionals to play a much greater role in defining quality goals and other objectives in the delivery of medical care. If the medical profession is to maintain its power to shape its own identity, it will need to ensure that it remains involved in developing regulatory tools.

This chapter explores the challenges that the evolution in quality regulation presents for medical professionalism. It begins by describing the existing framework for quality regulation.[3] It explains how the information revolution has transformed quality regulation and what this transformation may mean for the delivery of medical care. It then discusses the difficulties involved in defining and fulfilling the professional responsibilities created by the spread of new quality tools. Finally, it analyzes the implications of regulatory evolution for the future of the medical profession.

The Nature of Quality Regulation

"Regulation" usually refers to government-imposed mandates, but this definition captures only a subset of the measures that influence the provision of medical care. This chapter defines regulation more broadly as all measures undertaken by third parties to influence the quality of specific providers,[4] regardless of whether the third parties are governmental or non-governmental, and regardless of whether the measures are rules, incentives, or other approaches to improving quality.

Regulatory measures fitting this broad definition take several forms, each with a different approach to influencing quality, and each with different consequences for individual patients.[5] The professional licensure process is the best example of classic, market-displacing regulation. Not just anyone can hang up a doctor's shingle. State statutes require prospective physicians to meet minimum requirements with respect to education, training, and testing. These statutes improve quality by precluding the delivery of care by those most likely to injure patients. By removing transactions between unlicensed providers and patients from the marketplace, this market-displacing form of regulation will tend to raise the minimum level of quality of care delivered. Licensure statutes benefit patients who would prefer to avoid care from providers who fall below the minimum quality threshold set by regulatory authorities, but who lack the information necessary to discern the identity of such physicians.

An alternative form of quality regulation supplies the information needed to avoid low-quality care, rather than attempting to eliminate low-quality care directly. This regulatory approach facilitates the operations of health care markets by remedying the information failures that prevent markets from working efficiently. Market-facilitating regulations, like market-displacing regulations, may result in the elimination of low-quality care, but only if those purchasing care choose to avoid lower-quality providers. More generally, market-facilitating regulations affect quality by influencing purchaser decision making. If the regulations are successful in addressing information and rationality deficiencies, and no other market imperfections exist, the distribution of quality in the health care marketplace will reflect purchasers' actual demand for quality. Market-facilitating quality regulations include reporting programs that disseminate information about health care quality to patients, as well as efforts to regulate the collection and analysis of data that underlie quality measures.

A third approach to quality regulation, the market-channeling approach, falls somewhere in-between market-displacing and market-facilitating approaches. Regulatory measures adopting this approach are not fully market-displacing, since they do not necessarily preclude patient access to particular providers; they are not purely market-facilitating, either, because the role of the third party regulator extends beyond simply providing information that patients can use in selecting providers. Market-channeling regulators improve quality by using their influence to alter providers' behavior in ways they think appropriate, rather than by prohibiting market transactions or eliminating information failures. Accreditation or board certification organizations, for example, are market-channeling because the criteria they select for the evaluation process are likely to influence provider behavior, regardless of whether a particular patient is aware of or concerned about the criteria. Pay-for-performance programs, under which payers offer financial rewards to providers for high-quality care,[6] also constitute market-channeling regulation. Payers, rather than individual patients, determine the criteria by which providers will be rewarded or penalized; they can encourage provider activities, including quality improvement, regardless of which activities a particular patient values.

Information-Driven Evolution of Quality Regulation

These three types of regulation can and do coexist, but their relative contributions to the overall regulatory framework have changed over time. In recent years, market-facilitating and market-channeling regulations have played increasingly important roles in influencing quality. This regulatory evolution is driven in significant part by advances in information technology.

Over the last several decades, technological innovations have greatly decreased the costs of collecting, processing, storing, evaluating, and disseminating information. Computers make possible the rapid aggregation and analysis of vast quantities of data; along with the Internet, they also facilitate sharing the results of any analyses with specific groups of people or with the public as a whole. In theory, these cost reductions could lessen the need for quality regulation. If patients could without cost acquire, analyze, and act upon accurate information about provider quality, there would be less to be gained from excluding some providers from the market. In practice, however, technological innovation has reduced but not eliminated information costs. Rather than obviate the need for quality regulation, innovation affects the relative importance of different types of regulation in the regulatory mix.

Information is a key input into the regulatory process. Physician licensure and credentialing, for example, rely on information about physician education and training and physician discipline; health care quality report cards and pay-for-performance programs rely on information about the health care delivery process and patient outcomes. Some of these types of information have been more affected by the information revolution than others. Information about physician education and training, for example, is fairly straightforward to collect and use. Computerization may have reduced the cost of storing and processing licensure information, but probably not by much relative to a pen-and-paper world. On the other hand, the health care process and outcome measures upon which many report cards and pay-for-performance programs depend would be quite costly in a world without computers. If our willingness to implement regulations depends at least in part on regulatory costs, then by reducing the costs of collecting, analyzing, and disseminating data, the information revolution should promote the growth of these information-intensive regulations relative to their less information-intensive counterparts.[7]

Changes in the regulatory framework have already begun, consistent with these predictions. While traditional market-displacing regulations remain in place, information-intensive regulations have proliferated. Motivated in part by renewed concern about rising health care costs and quality deficiencies, both public and private regulators have implemented market-facilitating and market-channeling regulatory approaches across the United States.

The trend toward publication of provider report cards is perhaps the most visible example of the expansion of market-facilitating regulation. Numerous entities have embraced this regulatory approach.[8] With respect to hospital services, for example, a federal government Web site publishes hospital-specific heart attack and heart failure mortality rates as well as measures of adherence to recommended practices for cardiac care, pneumonia care, and the prevention of surgical infections.[9] In Pennsylvania, an independent state agency publishes individual hospitals' and physicians' risk-adjusted mortality and readmission rates for cardiac bypass surgery as well as various quality measures for hip and knee replacements.[10] New York, New Jersey, and Texas, among other states, also publish hospital report cards.[11] Public entities continue to launch health care reporting efforts; Florida created its hospital comparison Web site in 2005,[12] for example, while in 2006, Colorado enacted legislation requiring report card publication.[13] In addition, in the last few years, many states have mandated the publication of hospital-specific data on hospital-acquired infections; in 2006, both Missouri[14] and Pennsylvania[15] began publishing this data.

Private entities such as accreditation organizations, health plans, and employers have begun to disseminate health care quality information as well. The Joint Commission, which accredits hospitals, publishes individual hospital quality data on a publicly accessible Web site.[16] The Leapfrog Group, whose membership includes health plans and employers, provides quality measures for hospitals nationwide based on their adoption of computerized order entry systems, intensive care unit staffing patterns, treatment patterns and performance, and safety practices.[17] A coalition of providers, insurers, employers, and others have developed a California hospital report card.[18] Health plans are also creating Web sites that provide information about health care quality to their enrollees.[19]

Many entities also publish information on *physician* quality. In the public sector, the most common type of physician quality information is based on data provided to state medical boards. For example, the Massachusetts Board of Registration in Medicine physician profile Web site provides information about the education, training, disciplinary history, and malpractice payment history of Massachusetts physicians.[20] Many other states provide similar information.[21]

Published assessments of the quality of physician services are less widespread. Pennsylvania and New York have taken the lead among public entities in publishing physician-specific data on health care outcomes; each provides surgeon-specific quality ratings based on risk-adjusted mortality rates for cardiac bypass surgery patients.[22] California has taken a different approach, publishing report cards on medical groups based on criteria such as immunization rates, screening practices, and patient satisfaction.[23] Private organizations have established quality reporting mechanisms as well; for example, in 2006 a Massachusetts coalition of providers, purchasers, consumers, and others created a Web site that offers information about the quality of care delivered by medical groups.[24] Health plans may also provide their members with information about physician quality.[25] The federal government does not yet publish physician quality data, but in 2007 it launched the Physician Quality Reporting Initiative, under which it began to collect data on quality from individual physicians.[26]

Like report card programs, pay-for-performance programs have spread rapidly in the information age. Employers and health plans participating in the national Bridges to Excellence program pay bonuses to physicians who satisfy a number of quality criteria, such as maintaining electronic medical records or meeting performance standards with respect to blood pressure.[27] Under the

California-based Integrated Healthcare Association program, health plans collectively covering millions of enrollees pay physician groups a bonus based on measures of clinical quality of care, patient satisfaction, and the use of information technology.[28] A study of more than 250 HMOs across the country found that over half included pay-for-performance mechanisms in their provider contracts.[29] State Medicaid programs have implemented pay-for-performance programs that reward physicians based on criteria such as the provision of screening and preventive services.[30] Medicare has undertaken multiple pay-for-performance demonstration projects,[31] and the Medicare Payment Advisory Commission has recommended that Medicare incorporate financial incentives for quality in its provider payment mechanisms.[32] While Medicare has not yet done so, it recently took steps to avoid paying for poor-quality care; it issued a rule denying payment for hospital care associated with certain types of preventable hospital-acquired conditions, such as some kinds of infections, pressure ulcers, and serious preventable events.[33]

Challenges of Regulatory Evolution for Medical Professionals

If the only effect of the information revolution were to improve existing regulation by making it cheaper or more precise, then medical professionals could respond simply by cheering it on. But because the information revolution is changing the mix of regulatory approaches, and because these regulatory approaches remain imperfect, they pose considerable challenges to physicians seeking to serve their patients' interests. By altering the way that health care quality is monitored, assessed, and allocated, regulatory evolution requires physicians to take on new responsibilities. Taking on new responsibilities is, of course, always a challenge, particularly for physicians who may already be overburdened. But before physicians can even begin to confront this challenge, they must take on another one: understanding the contours of these responsibilities.

Determining how physicians should respond to new regulatory developments is difficult in part because of the lack of a single source of governing principles for medical professionals. Moreover, even with an authoritative document, most articulations of professional obligations are too general to offer concrete guidance about how to respond in particular situations. In addition, even general professionalism principles often point in different directions, a problem rooted in the complexity of professionals' roles in society.

Absent space for a comprehensive survey and analysis in this chapter, we will make do by using as a guide the most comprehensive recent conception of medical professionalism: the Physician Charter developed by the American Board of Internal Medicine Foundation, the American College of Physicians-American

Society of Internal Medicine Foundation, and the European Federation of Internal Medicine.[34] The charter, like most of its predecessors and competitors, identifies three fundamental principles of medical professionalism: the primacy of patient welfare, respect for patient autonomy, and the need to promote social justice.[35] We examine the implications of each of these three principles for the nature of physicians' obligations in an information-rich age.

Patient Welfare

An obvious professional obligation to arise out of the information revolution is to use these new tools to improve quality of care. The primacy of patient welfare imposes on physicians a responsibility to seek quality improvement. To the extent that the information revolution might make possible alternative, better mechanisms for quality improvement, physicians have an obligation to explore them. The charter makes this obligation explicit in its "commitment to improving quality of care":

> Physicians must actively participate in the development of better measures of quality of care and the application of quality measures to assess routinely the performance of all individuals, institutions, and systems responsible for health care delivery. Physicians . . . must take responsibility for assisting in the creation and implementation of mechanisms designed to encourage continuous improvement in the quality of care.[36]

But what does "actively participate" and "assist in" entail? Professional principles provide little guidance. At a minimum, physicians should not actively subvert quality improvement initiatives by refusing to participate. But how much more should physicians do to advance patient welfare?

Beyond simply not subverting quality measures, physicians can use performance or quality measures to improve patient well-being in many ways. They can implement or participate in programs to collect data on quality. They can review quality measures generated by internal data collection systems, public report cards, or pay-for-performance programs in order to determine whether changes in their delivery of care might be warranted. They can use information on quality to evaluate the comparative strengths of hospitals or specialists to which they might refer a patient. And, if patients arrive with incomplete or incorrect information they have found on their own, physicians can work to set them straight.

They can also work to improve the quality of quality measures. Imperfect quality improvement initiatives may actually create incentives that worsen care, by encouraging providers to avoid patients[37] or conditions they fear will lower quality scores.[38] The incentive to avoid patients who are more likely to produce lower quality scores can be mitigated if quality measures are improved, which itself requires active physician participation in developing and validating quality measures. Accordingly, numerous state and specialty medical societies have joined with federal agencies and other organizations to create and disseminate quality measures through the American Medical Association–convened Physician Consortium for Performance Improvement.[39] The consortium developed nearly 80 percent of the measures included in Medicare's 2007 Physician Quality Reporting Initiative.[40]

Furthermore, physicians can take advantage of quantitative measures of quality to improve regulatory systems of all kinds. As Timothy Jost has argued, for example, medical boards should investigate providers who perform especially poorly on performance measures.[41] The importance of physician involvement in collection and use of performance measures has already been recognized by some specialty boards, including the American Board of Internal Medicine, which has incorporated the use of performance data into their certification processes.[42]

The list of potential professional obligations could extend even further. For example, one might argue that physicians should adopt information systems that would facilitate their participation in quality measurement programs. Electronic medical records would likely increase the accuracy of data underlying these measures, make feasible the collection of a broader set of quality measures, and improve the risk adjustment algorithms necessary to make quality measures reliable. A 2005 survey, however, suggested that only about one quarter of office-based physicians used electronic medical record systems.[43] Clearly, physicians could build a better foundation for performance measures by contributing to discussions about electronic medical record design, increasing use of electronic systems, participating in efforts to construct data sharing frameworks, and building support for the wide data sharing needed to produce databases of sufficient size to create meaningful quality measures.[44] One is hard pressed to argue, however, that adopting state-of-the-art information systems is mandated by the Physician Charter's general exhortations.

Patient Autonomy

The Physician Charter identifies patient autonomy as the second of three fundamental principles of medical professionalism, and states that physicians must "empower" patients "to make informed decisions about their treatment."[45] The charter also articulates a commitment to honesty with patients, under which physicians should inform patients about error-induced injuries and "must ensure that patients are completely and honestly informed before the patient has consented to treatment."[46]

These provisions contemplate information sharing about a treatment under consideration, such as its likely benefits and risks. The information revolution, however, may alter the nature of information appropriately shared with patients. The more data that is available, the more precise the information physicians will be able to provide about benefits and risks of treatment in a particular context. But how much information must a physician provide for a patient to be "completely and honestly informed" and "empowered"? Taking the time to do this with each patient to the fullest extent possible will reduce the time available to pursue many other important and welfare-enhancing goals in a medical encounter, such as counseling patients about various ways to promote health and prevent disease, or doing a more thorough assessment of psychosocial factors that contribute to a patient's condition.

Even with sufficient time, there are limits to what professional rules realistically can expect of ordinary mortals. Imagine, for instance, a competent but relatively inexperienced surgeon or one whose track record is adequate but worse than average. Does professionalism require that surgeons tell their patients about their less-than-stellar individual qualifications or track records for proposed treatments?

While the Physician Charter does not answer this specific question, courts have confronted similar questions in cases alleging violations of informed consent. In a case involving a surgeon who chose to present risks in statistical terms and misled his patient about his experience, the court suggested that informed consent might sometimes require disclosure of a physician's level of experience, the risks of treatment adjusted for physician experience, and the availability of lower-risk surgery elsewhere.[47] However, other courts have proved more reluctant to expand informed consent obligations to include information about lack of surgical experience[48] or other provider-specific characteristics. Despite the undeniable materiality of such information, courts have expressed concern that requiring physician-specific risk disclosures would raise an impracticable impediment to the efficient rendering of professional services[49] and would lead to endless and unpredictable demands for "every fact which might conceivably affect performance in the surgical suite,"[50] including medical school grades,[51] whether the doctor had a good marriage,[52] and whether he or she slept well the night before surgery.[53] Similar questions about where to draw the line complicate efforts to interpret the professional obligations to protect autonomy and ensure honesty. If report card scores predict outcomes better than medical school grades, one might try to argue for drawing the line between the two, requiring disclosure of the former but not the latter. On the other hand, even limited disclosure requirements could burden the treatment relationship.

A second area of relevant legal precedent involves informing patients of limitations set by managed care plans. When health insurers restrict what they pay for, or when they reward physicians for saving health care costs, they create a potential conflict of interest between the patient's welfare and the physician's finances. Standard professional and legal principles require that patients be informed of this potential conflict so they can consider it in deciding how best to interact with their physicians. Yet, law and ethics have stopped short of requiring that physicians make such disclosures at the point of each treatment decision. Courts have been reluctant to impose liability on physicians for failing to disclose managed care restrictions.[54]

In practice, the few physicians who disclose potential managed care-related conflicts of interest tend not to do so "at the bedside." Their clinics give new patients a brochure that describes financial and contractual arrangements with health plans.[55] Disclosures about potential conflicts of interest are more often made by health plans prior to treatment, as part of insurance enrollment. Similarly, in the report card context, it may make more sense for physicians to meet the challenge of fulfilling professional obligations to protect patient autonomy not through discussions about ratings at the bedside, but instead by publicizing the availability of report cards for patient use. Moreover, the availability of report cards through managed care and public Web sites may reduce the need for physicians to counsel patients about the report cards' contents.

In short, while disclosing quality information is sometimes appropriate—the most obvious case being a physician's disclosure of quality information about a provider the physician recommends—professionalism may not require universal disclosure of report card information during the course of the treatment relationship. While fuller disclosure may promote patient autonomy, it may ultimately compete with the professional obligation to serve patient welfare. As the California Supreme Court observed in *Arato v. Avedon*, "[t]he [clinical contexts] in which physicians and patients interact and exchange information . . . are so multifarious, the information needs and degree of dependency of individual patients so various, and the professional relationship itself such an intimate and irreducibly judgment-laden one, that we believe it is unwise to require as a matter of law that a particular species of information be disclosed."[56]

Social Justice

The Physician Charter's third fundamental principle is that of social justice, which requires promoting the "fair distribution of health care resources" as well as eliminating discrimination based on race, gender, socioeconomic status, or other illegitimate characteristics.[57] Similarly, the charter's commitment to improving access to care states that physicians "should work to eliminate barriers to access based on education, laws, finances, geography, and social discrimination."[58] It adds that "[m]edical professionalism demands that the objective of all health care systems be the availability of a uniform and adequate standard of care."[59]

Of all the obligations recognized by the charter, the pursuit of social justice is the one that poses the most significant challenge for physicians in the new information age. Altering the mix of regulations to include more market-facilitating and market-channeling approaches to regulation may lead to greater dispersion in standards of care and greater disparities in delivery of care.[60]

Traditional market-displacing health care quality regulations such as licensure do not necessarily ensure uniformity in the quality of care. Instead, they tend to compress the distribution of quality by eliminating what would otherwise be the lowest-quality providers. Within the remaining distribution of quality, they do nothing to upset the existing allocation of quality. In other words, some patients receive higher-quality services, and others lower-quality services; market-displacing minimum quality regulations do nothing to affect who receives what sort of care, as long as the regulation-defined minimum is met.[61] In a world with limited information, clinical quality might be allocated randomly across patients because patients are not able to differentiate better from worse physicians.

By contrast, market-facilitating regulations may allocate high-quality care according to criteria that some may find objectionable, such as ability to pay. In a perfectly competitive world consisting only of patients and physicians, patients would use the quality information to seek out the highest-quality physicians. Competition would push down fees paid to lower-quality physicians and encourage other physicians to increase their quality. Unlike market-displacing regulations, however, market-facilitating regulations do not necessarily eliminate low-quality care; they permit and even encourage variations in quality, to the extent that market participants seek different levels of quality. Some patients end up purchasing the services of lower-quality providers, either because they are less concerned about quality differentials or because they lack financial resources. The prospect that wealthier patients may systematically receive a higher quality of care will trouble those who believe that social justice requires uniformity, but the charter itself does not insist on strict uniformity. Instead, it hedges by calling for the "availability" of a "uniform and adequate" standard of care.

Some forces may dampen the influence of patient income on the allocation of care. Most obviously, if quality competition fails to take hold because patients ignore report card results, then report cards would be unlikely to strengthen the connection between willingness to pay and higher-quality care. Moreover, if insurers maintain broad networks that include physicians of varying quality and decline to pass along quality-related fee differentials to their enrollees, then patients will be less likely to be matched to physicians based on the patients' financial resources. In addition, to the extent that physicians pursue high quality and are similarly equipped to achieve it, competition may not produce quality differentiation sufficient to be tracked by report cards. Ultimately, however, if quality differentials remain and report cards publicize them, access to high-quality care is likely to be in part a function of patient income.

Equally troubling is that quality reporting may widen health care disparities along non-financial dimensions. If ratings are not fully risk-adjusted, physicians may be able to increase their scores by avoiding patients who are more severely ill. Even adequate risk adjustors may produce this behavior if physicians still believe that the risk adjustment mechanism is insufficient. Either through perception or through reality, inadequate risk adjustment will generate disparities in access to treatment and potentially in treatment outcomes based on the severity of the patients' underlying illness. The most severely ill may be deprived of access to care they would have received in a regulatory framework dominated by more traditional market-displacing forms of regulation.

Quality reporting's challenge for social justice does not end there. If physicians cannot determine the severity of patients' illnesses, they may discriminate based on factors they believe are associated with severity, producing disparities along other dimensions. Similar disparities may result from quality measures that are affected by patient behaviors. For instance, if physicians believe that some groups, such as members of racial minorities or the less well educated, are less likely to adhere to medical recommendations,[62] then they may discriminate on that basis.[63] If so, reporting will increase racial disparities.

Early studies of bypass surgery report cards suggest that there is reason to be concerned about these selection effects. One study found that in states with public report cards the composition of bypass surgery patients shifted toward more healthy patients.[64] Another study found an initial increase in disparities in bypass surgery rates between white patients, on the one hand, and black and

Hispanic patients, on the other, immediately after New York's publication of bypass surgery report cards.[65] These studies indicate that physicians may respond to reporting programs by altering their selection of patients. Depending on the form it takes, this sort of gaming has the potential to increase access barriers, exacerbate treatment disparities, and worsen health care outcomes. It is therefore inconsistent with the obligations of medical professionalism.[66]

Gaming is not the only potential cause of reporting-related health care disparities, however. Even if report cards are properly risk adjusted, disparities may result from differentials in report cards' use. The patients most likely to benefit from quality reporting are those who read report cards and then use the information to select high-quality providers. Not everyone seeks out quality information. One 2006 survey found that about 29 percent of respondents used the Internet to search for information about a particular doctor or hospital.[67] Another 2006 survey found that about 20 percent of respondents had used quality information to make health care decisions; about 12 percent of respondents saw information specifically about physicians, and over half of these respondents used it.[68] These statistics suggest that quality reporting is an important tool for many patients, but that many others still do not consult report cards before making decisions about their care.

The information revolution is most likely to leave behind patients for whom information is difficult to acquire or use.[69] One type of barrier is technological. Because a significant proportion of quality information is available through the Internet, patients who lack Internet access will face more difficulty in searching for high-quality providers than those who have high-speed Internet access from home.[70] Respondents to a 2006 survey who were older, lower-income, less well educated, women, black, or lived in rural areas were less likely to be Internet users than their counterparts, and so less likely to benefit from quality reporting mechanisms.[71] In addition, among those with Internet access, some groups, such as younger patients and better educated patients, were disproportionately more likely to use report cards to search for information about particular providers.[72]

These demographic differences may be in part a function of differences in the groups' abilities to take full advantage of the information available in report cards. Those who are poorly educated, have limited literacy, speak languages other than English, or suffer from diminished cognitive capacity may find themselves unable to understand report card contents, particularly when the report cards provide overly detailed information about specific conditions.[73] The most severely ill are also likely to face great difficulty in using report cards, either because of diminished cognitive or physical abilities, or because

their emotional state prevents rational consideration of report card information. Those who do not understand report cards may decline to use them, or
even worse, use them improperly, so that they select poorer rather than higher-
quality providers. In short, quality reporting may increase disparities between
patients who are well equipped to make use of report cards and those who
are not.[74]

Patients need not use report cards to benefit from them. If enough potential
patients use report cards to select providers, then physicians may have an
incentive to increase quality for all of their patients, even if a subset are unaware
of the report cards' existence. However, some physicians inevitably will have
patients who, overall, are more responsive to these competitive forces than
other physicians' patients. For example, report cards are more likely to accelerate competition among physicians practicing in areas dominated by more highly
educated and better-insured patients. They are also more likely to be effective
in urban areas, where patients have more provider choices than in rural areas.
If physicians' potential patient populations vary in propensity to use report
cards, then physicians' responsiveness to report cards is likely to vary as well,
potentially increasing disparities.

Market-channeling regulatory approaches pose a different set of challenges
for social justice. Like market-facilitating regulations, they contemplate a full
range of provider quality levels; they do not preclude access to low-quality
providers. The feature that distinguishes them from market-facilitating regulations is their dependence on third-party channeling entities, such as insurers
or medical specialty boards. Knowledgeable third parties can create quality
improvement mechanisms that protect patients without regard to patients' ability to comprehend report cards or to act as savvy consumers in the marketplace.
A medical specialty board, for example, may partly serve a market-facilitating
function in that it communicates to patients an assessment of provider quality through the board certification process. However, it also serves a channeling function by selecting particular quality criteria to judge physicians, thus
encouraging physicians to take the steps necessary to meet these criteria. Patients
need not be aware of these criteria to benefit from them. Similarly, pay-for-
performance programs encourage physicians to improve their delivery of care
even if their patients are unaware of the programs' existence. Because channeling approaches do not depend on patients' use of information, they will not
produce disparities in the same way that report cards do.

Market-channeling regulations may still have implications for social justice, however. First, like report cards, market-channeling regulations can generate disparities if the quality measures they rely on function poorly. Second,

market-channeling entities may serve limited populations. Providers who serve many patients whose insurers implement pay-for-performance programs, for example, will face different incentives than will providers who disproportionately serve the uninsured. Third, market-channeling regulations that tie pay to performance can exacerbate disparities by directing financial rewards to the providers who need them least. If engaging in quality improvement activities is expensive, then mechanisms that redirect funds from low-quality to high-quality practices will tend to dampen efforts to improve quality among those most in need of improvement. Note that if enrollees are aware of providers' quality ratings, they could avoid the negative consequences of this effect by simply switching providers. In reality, however, many enrollees will not be aware of their physicians' ratings or will be unable to switch for geographical or other reasons. This means that they may end up paying higher premiums to support pay-for-performance programs without getting better care.

In short, the expansion of market-facilitating and market-channeling regulations may raise social justice concerns articulated by the Physician Charter. But physicians can address these concerns.[75] They should support or help develop risk adjustment mechanisms that will combat the gaming that might otherwise occur in report card or pay-for-performance programs.[76] They should advocate for reimbursement mechanisms that reward not just high levels of quality, but also quality improvement, to ensure that funds flow to physician practices in need of improvement. Based on their experience in working with patients, they could suggest ways to make publicly reported measures easier to understand and use. Physicians could work with individual patients to help them overcome any barriers they may face in using report cards; for instance, when making referrals to specialists, they could alert patients to the availability of report cards and explain how to use them. Finally, physicians could respond to social justice concerns by bringing attention to them. For example, they could participate in studies of the effects of specific types of regulations on disparities and then use this information to advocate for the adoption, abandonment, or redesign of particular regulatory approaches.[77]

Implications of Regulatory Evolution
for the Future of the Medical Profession

Physicians have never been fans of regulation, but newer forms of regulation are seen by some as especially threatening to professional interests. The increasing emphasis on market competition might undermine the special relationships between professionals and their clients, threatening the very core of professionalism.[78] This view is shortsighted. In working to improve quality measures to achieve patient welfare and social justice goals, physicians would act in the interest of not just their patients, but also their profession.

Under the traditional market-displacing regulatory regimes such as licensure, it is largely physicians who set quality standards and determine whether they have been met. But under market-facilitating and market-channeling regulations, physicians cede to others some of their power to define standards. Under market-facilitating regulations, it is patients who decide which criteria to use in selecting their physicians. Under market-channeling regulations, the channeling entities shape standards; pay-for-performance programs, for example, give payers significant influence over the practices of physicians. In short, the information revolution gives non-physicians a large role to play in quality oversight.[79]

Some physicians have resisted the expansion of non-physicians' oversight roles through mechanisms such as pay-for-performance programs.[80] Given current patient, payer, and policymaker interest in these measures, however, the programs are likely to persist. Furthermore, the Physician Charter's commitment to "accepting external scrutiny of all aspects of . . . professional performance" suggests that physicians should support the development of such programs. By participating in the creation and review of quality measures, physicians can help to ensure that they accurately reflect quality and avoid unintended consequences for both patients and physicians.

Continued physician involvement in the development of performance measures is also important because it allows physicians to shape the nature of the regulatory influences they face and, more generally, the future of medical care. The information revolution facilitates the growth of market-facilitating and market-channeling mechanisms by permitting information to be collected, analyzed, and disseminated widely. But in order for this to happen, someone must determine what sorts of information to collect and what sorts of measures to compile. By retaining a voice in the creation of quality measures, physicians can exercise influence over the issues on which patients and third parties focus. Report cards allow patients to shape the nature of physicians' practices, for example, but only with respect to the issues covered by the report cards. Physicians can help determine which quality issues deserve the most attention.[81]

Skeptics might worry that heavy involvement of organized medicine in quality oversight will jeopardize the stringency of these measures. Despite this legitimate concern, physician involvement is better than forceful opposition by the medical establishment. Professional*ism* need not equate with professional *dominance*.[82] Guided by the charter's exhortations, physicians can play a constructive role both in crafting quality measures and in promoting their acceptance. In a world in which perfect quality measures are unlikely to be achieved, physicians can help determine which of the inevitable compromises are preferable.

Admittedly, there are many obstacles to greater physician involvement. While medical specialty societies would seem to have an important role to play in developing quality measures, a recent study suggests that only about a third of medical societies are currently involved in the process, for reasons that include member reluctance, limited resources, and the difficulty of obtaining consensus.[83] Many medical professionals lack the technical expertise necessary to participate fully in the design of quality measures,[84] so would need to acquire this expertise themselves or rely on others for it.

Given the high stakes for both physicians and their patients, however, medical organizations have reason to expand their involvement in these programs. By taking full advantage of the tools the information revolution makes possible, physicians can meet the challenge of advancing the core values of medical professionalism while simultaneously advancing the interests of the profession.

The "Information Rx"

In October 2007, Zagat Survey LLC, the company long known for its popular restaurant and hotel guides, announced a new venture: a Zagat's guide to doctors. In collaboration with WellPoint Inc., the nation's largest health insurance company, Zagat began in January 2008 to do online surveys with select patients. Following the same format developed for its other guides, Zagat's collected information about patients' satisfaction with their physicians on four criteria—trust, communication, availability, and office environment—and used them to rank doctors on a thirty-point scale. As Nina Zagat, the company's co-founder, explained, "With this tool, WellPoint is helping to give consumers the power to make smart decisions about selecting doctors based on other people's experiences." Eric Fennel, WellPoint's vice president of consumer innovation, echoed her enthusiasm, saying that such "peer-to-peer information" constituted "the missing piece of information needed to engage consumers" and provided a much needed adjunct to the "clinical and cost information" that the company already provided its enrollees.[1]

Zagat's entry into the doctor rating field prompted a range of responses from the amused to the skeptical. "Would you like dessert with your diagnosis?" one headline read, while another announced "the time is coming when you can pick up the 'burgundy bible' to find the best restaurant in town, and then search a similar guide to find a gastroenterologist to treat the possible stomach ache afterwards." Not surprisingly, physician reaction to rankings based on patient satisfaction was at best lukewarm. The response from James King, the president of the American Academy of Family Physicians, was typical: He warned that "choosing a physician only according to consumer ratings can deprive patients of high quality medical care, particularly if those ratings are based on unrecognized and unvoiced anger or unjustified allegiance."[2]

But in spite of such warnings, the enthusiasm for consumer-oriented rankings, report cards, and other information tools reflected in the Zagat's guide seems here to stay in the United States. Besides the Zagat/WellPoint survey, patients can now go online to sites such as Rate MD.com, Vitals.com, and DrScore.com to share their opinions about specific doctors. These so called peer-to-peer evaluations join a field already crowded by other types of information sources intended to help patients make better choices. Some focus on therapeutic issues (is this the best treatment or hospital for me?); others concentrate on cost effectiveness (is this the most economical use of my health care dollar?)

While measuring very different phenomena—subjective measures of trust as well as seemingly more objective measures of therapeutic success or fiscal prudence—these consumer information sources all purport to be a more neutral, reliable sort of information than the paltry sources available to patients in the past. In tandem with similar efforts aimed at better assessing physician performance through supposedly objective measures of quality and cost effectiveness, better forms of information technology are frequently hailed as a promising new direction in health care reform. As *USA Today* observed in a 2008 article on the Zagat/Wellpoint venture, "medicine is just the latest profession to feel the Internet's power to gather information and disseminate it to consumers hungry for the best service or value, and it's going to have to adapt as the others did."[3]

Underlying faith in this "information Rx"—that is, the belief that providing more and better information to individual consumers can reform the American health care system—is the related assumption that the health care market needs to become more like other aspects of the American economy. If only consumers had access to the same quantity and quality of information available for goods such as appliances or automobiles, so the argument goes, they could be a powerful force for improvement in health care. As one commentator put it, "if Zagat's can rate Chinese restaurants and Greek tavernas, and *Consumer Reports* can rate skateboards and digital cameras, why can't we rate doctors?" With better information about physicians, hospitals, and insurance plans, Regina Herzlinger, Michael L. Millenson, and others have argued, consumers will reward the good and avoid the bad, thereby turning the power of individual choice into a powerful tool of change.[4]

This conception of an information-driven consumer health "revolution" exemplifies two important trends of the last forty years: the reliance on market forces to reform an ailing health care system and the enthusiasm for computer-assisted information technologies, including but by no means limited to the Internet. The proliferation of decision making tools nowadays offered the afflu-ent American patient/consumer illustrates the strong faith in what art historian Theodore Roszak has referred to as the "godword" of information, a once "non-descript word rarely used for anything more exalted than requesting a tele-phone number ('Information, please')" that in his words now enjoys "the mystique once reserved for Reason, Faith, [and] Grace."[5]

The information Rx, as well as the larger field of quality assessment upon which it rests, has gained this exalted status for many reasons. The idea of the informed patient/consumer reflects a venerable American tradition of relying on individual education as a tool of personal and collective change. Informed patient choice seemingly applies to medicine the same processes that have worked to improve other sectors of the American economy over the last cen-tury. The emphasis on individual preference is particularly well suited to the decentralized, "marketized" health care system that has evolved in the United States since the 1970s. Last, but not least, more and better consumer informa-tion is one of the few policy goals on which liberals and conservatives have consistently been able to agree since the 1970s.[6]

The political appeal and ideological expediency of the information Rx makes it all the more difficult to question its value. Yet question it we must, for informed policy discussion requires taking a long hard look at its utility. Other chapters in this volume ask hard questions about the implications of new infor-mation technologies for physicians and other health care decision makers. This chapter focuses on the perceived link between consumer empowerment and information access. My intention here is not to discredit the idea that con-sumers deserve good information, a principle that it is hard to dispute, but rather to raise more basic questions about what constitutes "good" information, in the hope of encouraging a more realistic appreciation of what the consumer information Rx can—and cannot—accomplish.

My argument here employs what, at first glance, may seem like an irrele-vant or inappropriate methodology, namely historical analysis. One of the most common assumptions about the modern information revolution is that it is without historical precedent. The Zagat's guide, and all it represents (e.g., patients using the Internet, consumers "driving" the health care market) are invariably presented as the innovation without precedent, the "something new under the sun," that has no history. To the historian (or at least this historian) that kind of claim is like catnip to a cat, or red meat to a dog: it is an assertion that begs for contradiction.

Hence the purpose of this chapter is to sketch the history of buying guides, report cards, and other rating devices aimed at patient/consumers. It attempts to put the brave new world of the modern health consumer exemplified by the Zagat's guide, and its many competitors and imitators, into long range historical perspective. By tracing the evolution of arguments linking consumer empowerment with new information technology, I hope to accomplish three goals: first, to counter simplistic historical narratives that overemphasize the role of the Internet as the starting point of such developments; second, to complicate the meaning of "consumer information" as a keyword frequently invoked in health policy debates; and third, to highlight the changing, often contradictory meanings of expertise and the question of who "owns" it, as they have evolved over the last half century. As we shall see, the "information Rx" has been not unlike the modern prescription drug: highly effective in correcting an underlying pathology, but accompanied by unexpected side effects. A better understanding of its benefits and risks may help to improve the next generation of remedies.

Report Cards and Buying Guides: Definitions and Origins

My argument here builds on a broader scholarly effort to put the late twentieth-century "information age" into historical perspective. I am particularly interested in exploring the ways that the creation and popularization of ranking measures help to create the very object they purport to study, as Wendy Espeland, Michael Sauder, Sarah Igo, and others have demonstrated so well in their work. As Espeland and Sauder have written, rankings and ratings "serve to recreate social worlds." In the same spirit, I seek to explore how new forms of consumer health information have helped to create and define the very concept of the modern health consumer. As such, consumer guides to health care constitute a very revealing "technology of knowledge," that is, a means of collecting and organizing information toward a specific end, in this case improvement of a health care service or institution.[7]

Consumer ratings and rankings depend for their utility on an easily quantifiable and understandable metric: the numbers conveyed are usually simple descriptive statistics, such as percentages, which are harnessed to a system of grading, ranging from excellent to unacceptable. Their construction requires the identification of a limited set of qualities or conditions to be measured, such as mortality rates or post operative infections; these benchmarks stand in for a more global assessment of performance or value too time-consuming to conduct. While producing a rating may require many hours of complex data analysis, the final form is still minimalist in its presentation. The user need not appreciate multivariate statistics or measures of statistical significance in order to comprehend the results.

Since the 1970s, computer-assisted technologies have made it far easier to compile ratings and rankings, and thus their appearance is often assumed to be a direct effect of the computer revolution. But as Daniel Headrick, Theodore Porter, and other historians have noted, modern information systems originated long before the computer. The predecessors of the modern consumer guide were technologies of knowledge produced by simple hand tabulations and statistical expressions. Moreover, the appeal of the technologies of knowledge today depends in no small part on their similarity to older forms of ranking and rating with which average Americans have long been familiar.[8]

That connection is evident in the frequent use of the term "report card" to encompass the new consumer-oriented information courses on offer today. The report card was a historical product of the American public school system. The first report cards developed as part of Progressive Era educational reform, which created age-specific grades as a way to standardize and improve the quality of the public school system. Starting as simple records of attendance and test performance, school report cards quickly expanded to include health and conduct issues as well.[9] In this era, reformers conceived of the disciplinary effect of the report card as going in one direction, namely to judge the pupil. But the potential existed to "turn the tables" so to speak, that is, to hold the teacher responsible for the students' failure to perform well.

Although they did not refer to them as "report cards," nineteenth-century health care reformers utilized similar methods. The contemporary quality assessment movement traces its origins to the work of Florence Nightingale, who collected and analyzed mortality statistics as a means to compel hospital reform in late nineteenth-century London. Using statistical data to measure and improve public health measures also found many adherents in the United States. Collection of mortality (and later morbidity) data became the foundation for discussions about the state of the nation's health.[10]

The convergence of Progressive Era educational and health care reform resulted in one of the most influential grading exercises of the twentieth century, namely the landmark 1910 Flexner Report. With funding from the Carnegie Foundation, Abraham Flexner and his associates created a medical school "report card" based on bench-marks that they felt captured the quality of a medical education; for example, what percentage of students had a college degree before entering, how many professors were full-time instructors, and how much time students spent in bedside instruction. By taking the Johns Hopkins model of medical education as its gold standard, the Flexner reforms devised a ranking system that helped close down "inferior" schools, including those serving women and blacks. From start to finish, this system of reviewing medical schools was conceived of as a dispassionate review by educational experts for educational experts, and not as a democratic form of information sharing, a point to which I will return below.[11]

During the same time period, the Boston surgeon Ernest Amory Codman developed an equally ambitious plan to assess the quality of hospitals and physicians' services. Like Nightingale, Codman is today venerated as a modern pioneer of quality improvement, but in his own time, his call to monitor the outcomes of hospital treatment aroused considerable resistance. (He anticipated that his epitaph would read, "EAC—killed by his colleagues.") Although less immediately influential than Flexner's report, Codman's "end results system" did influence the voluntary hospital accreditation program developed by the American College of Surgeons.[12]

In time, hospital accreditation became as important an assessment tool as the credentialing of medical schools. After the failure of New Deal efforts to enact a national health insurance program, hospital expansion, as funded by the landmark 1946 Hill-Burton Act, became the chief means to improve access to and quality of care. As the postwar hospital building boom took off, accreditation assumed even more significance as a regulatory mechanism; in 1951, the Joint Commission on Accreditation of Hospitals (JCAH) was founded as an independent, nonprofit organization devoted solely to that purpose. Further expansions of the American health care system in the 1960s would be securely tied to the JCAH accreditation process.[13]

But it is important to emphasize here that, prior to the 1960s, these kinds of grading exercises figured *only* as tool of expert assessment and policy formation; they were meant to be compiled by experts, and used by experts. In this respect, accreditation reviews and rankings differed greatly from the student report card, a "technology of knowledge" explicitly designed to be shared with pupils and their parents. In contrast, the first health care report cards were *always* meant for limited consumption: they were meant to influence the stewards of the institution not its end users. In other words, Abraham Flexner did not intend the Flexner Report to be used by medical students looking for a good medical school, nor did the JCAH think of its accreditation ratings as being useful to patients looking for a good hospital. The limited accessibility of information about health care reflected the prevailing conviction that patients could never evaluate the true value of the medical care they received, but rather needed to rely on their doctors' guidance in making choices about treatment.

This "patients should be seen but not heard" attitude stood in marked contrast to a new conception of rational choice in the marketplace that developed in the larger economy. Starting in the Progressive Era, the idea of the educated consumer gained traction in many different areas starting with the safety of foods and medicines, as evidenced in the 1906 Pure Food and Drugs Act that created the Food and Drug Administration (FDA). During the same time period, the home economics movement taught American women to regard careful shopping habits as a badge of domestic virtue. As a mass consumer economy expanded in the first three decades of the twentieth century, this ideal of careful consumption spread along with it. The economic collapse that gave rise to the Great Depression only intensified the emphasis on the importance of wise buying habits.[14]

In this climate, a new kind of consumers' "buyers' guide" became popular in the 1930s. This new style buyers' guide represented a very different conception of expertise from that embodied in medical school and hospital accreditation. The Depression era buyers' guide offered what today is referred to as "peer-to-peer" evaluations; the end users of the product, also known as consumers, sought to share their knowledge with their fellow consumers. Positioning themselves as representatives of "the consumer," interwar consumer advocates began to generate their own estimates of the value and quality of mass produced consumer goods: they sought to gather "unbiased" information—by which they meant information not produced solely as puffery by the company making the product— about specific products: did they perform as advertised? Did they "wear" well?

This mentality emerged in the late 1920s within informal consumer clubs formed to discuss how to help middle-class Americans get their "money's worth" in a rapidly expanding, advertising saturated economy. As the Great Depression set in, these sorts of questions became even more pressing, leading to the creation of a new kind of consumer group: first represented by Consumers' Research (CR), founded in 1929, and later by its rival Consumers Union (CU) founded in 1935. (CU went on to found what in the 1970s became a highly successful empire of consumer guides represented by *Consumer Reports*.) These organizations tapped a lucrative and appreciative market for a more critical kind of consumers' buying guide that sought to test the validity of manufacturers' claims. In preparing such guides, CR and CU stressed their virtues as independent, not-for-profit organizations whose sole aim was protecting consumer interests. To this end, they pioneered new methods of product evaluation and testing that became the standard for industrial quality control. They also played up their refusal to accept any kind of advertising in their publications as proof of their commercial disinterestedness.

These early consumer buying guides focused on mass produced products, not professional services because the former was far easier to test and categorize. They also concentrated on product lines where consumers' preferences could more easily be studied. In light of the "patients should be seen and not heard" philosophy, their forays into health care concentrated chiefly on denouncing proprietary medicine companies and alternative medicine, positions that on the surface made their work compatible with that of the powerful American Medical Association (AMA). In private, the relations between the new consumer groups and the AMA were strained, and consumer advocates had much to say about the arrogance of the medical profession. But those views rarely made it into print. It was far safer to criticize the corporate behavior of the proprietary drug industry than it was to challenge the AMA. Hence the famous "guinea pig" books of the 1930s concentrated on food, drugs, and cosmetics, as did the articles appearing in the publications put out by CR and CU. The home medical guide, *Good Health and Bad Medicine*, written in 1940 by CU's staff physician, Harold Aaron, stuck to a simple rating of over the counter drugs as "acceptable" or "not acceptable."[15]

This cautious tone reflects the political difficulties encountered by early consumer organizations. In the 1930s, the idea of independent consumer evaluation of health care products and services was tinged with radicalism. As Lisabeth Cohen has shown, the idea of the consumer citizen was strongly associated with the New Deal; consumer groups fell afoul of the same currents of conservatism directed against the New Dealers. Starting in the 1930s, conservatives began to accuse consumer groups of being Communist sympathizers, accusations that only intensified during the Cold War. For different reasons, specialists in health care research and policy also scorned the early consumer groups' efforts, regarding their claims to expertise in evaluating products as unfounded. Still, the concept of the "consumer buying guide" found a receptive audience among middle-class Americans, particularly the college-educated and professional groups which had growing confidence in their own powers of judgment. After years of being issued report cards and encouraged to patronize accredited schools, affluent Americans were starting to turn the tables.[16]

Power to the Patient

The political and cultural upheavals of the 1960s created a far more hospitable climate for the concept of the educated health care consumer. The Civil Rights, antiwar, students', and women's movements combined to encourage a widespread questioning of authority, including that of professional experts who became suspect as agents of the "establishment." Activists singled out the medical profession and the hospital industry as particularly complicit in the maintenance of a repressive social order. To counter this repressive influence, they called for a more democratic model of decision making in which patients had more control over their own treatments. A common characteristic of the many patient advocacy groups that sprang up in the 1960s and 1970s was a shared faith that more democratic decision making required better information about health care providers, treatments, and institutions.

The tight link between empowerment and information is well illustrated in the work of Public Citizen, the consumer organization founded by Ralph Nader in 1971. This was one of the new breed of citizens' advocacy groups that Michael Pertschuk has christened "giant killers." Public Citizen sought to combine critical information gathering with effective political action. Health care was among its earliest objects of critical scrutiny, evident in the creation of the Health Research Group, headed by physician Sidney Wolfe, as the first of Public Citizen's specialized subunits. The Nader-inspired critique of American health care faulted both the medical profession and government regulatory agencies for failing to defend patients' interests. Consumer advocates argued that the expert groups supposedly acting as guardians of patients' welfare were in fact captives of powerful special interests, among them the American Medical Association, the hospital industry, and the pharmaceutical industry. To offset this influence, Americans needed to become more savvy health care consumers, a goal that Public Citizen sought to promote through its research-based advocacy.[17]

This research-based advocacy took many forms. Initially, Public Citizen publications simply compiled and analyzed evidence from government reports and publications. The information needed to critique policy decision making was there in plain sight. But as consumer advocates quickly realized, the kind of information that newly empowered patient-consumers might need to make informed personal choices was far less accessible. Creating bodies of data truly useful to individual consumers required a very different approach.

One such effort consisted of publishing a consumers' guide to local physicians in a particular area. Although medical societies had long made available lists of their member doctors, they resisted the sharing of more specific facts about fees and treatment philosophies. Consumer advocates regarded this refusal to share data as symptomatic of the profession's undemocratic tendencies. If patients were ever to get better treatment, this medical "monopoly" on information had to be challenged. To that end, activist groups took up the idea of publishing a more consumer-friendly guide to local physicians.

One of the most publicized such efforts took place in the early 1970s, when a group affiliated with Public Citizen compiled a directory of physicians in Prince George's County, in Maryland, near Washington, D.C. The directory did not try to rate physicians, but simply aimed at giving patients basic information about the person's practice, such as office hours and fee scales; in addition, the directory makers sought to find out if doctors were willing to prescribe contraception for unmarried women, a major political issue in the early 1970s. When the local medical society learned of the directory project, it told its members not to cooperate, arguing that it constituted a form of physician advertising, which was forbidden by the AMA code of ethics. Although some doctors defied the medical society and allowed their information to be published, the majority did not.

The media coverage of what was styled as a "David and Goliath" battle between the medical society and the consumer activists attracted the attention of staff at the Federal Trade Commission (FTC), which had become interested in advertising bans among professional groups. The Prince Georges' County directory incident helped inspire the FTC's 1975 lawsuit against the American Medical Association, which eventually led to a lifting of the AMA's historic ban on physician advertising. Ironically, consumers' requests for more information about physicians led to an increased volume of advertising, a good example of the unintended consequences of reform.[18]

Similar controversies surrounded the creation of the first self-styled "buyers' guide" to hospital care, which appeared around the same time as the Prince George's County directory. Again, the idea for such a guide came from a Nader protégé, in this case Herb Denenberg. A law professor at the University of Pennsylvania, Denenberg was appointed commissioner of public insurance for the state of Pennsylvania in 1971 by the newly elected Democratic Governor Milton Shapp, who wanted to make the state's department of insurance more protective of policy holders. As commissioner, Denenberg used his regulatory authority to force insurance companies to disclose more information to their policy holders, a stance that soon earned him the nickname "horrible Herb" among insurance executives.[19]

Like the Maryland activists, Denenberg adopted the concept of a "shoppers' guide" as a way to promote more informed consumer choice. During his term as commissioner, his office put out a series of such guides, including ones on automobile and life insurance. The first and most controversial of these new-style buyers' guides was the 1971 *Shopper's Guide to Hospitals in the Philadelphia Area*. Even more modest in appearance than the Prince George's

County directory, Denenberg's first shopper's guide consisted of a one-page foldout listing daily rates, bed capacities, and average length of stay, and included information on deficiencies, in particular the number of "unsafe beds," gleaned from a report produced by Pennsylvania's Department of Health Education. It is worth noting that the use of the word "unsafe" echoed Ralph Nader's famous 1965 book on the automobile industry, *Unsafe at Any Speed*.[20]

But while limited in scope, the Philadelphia shoppers' guide to hospitals marked a dramatic change in policy philosophy. As Denenberg explained in his foreword, "Much of this information is supposed to be public information, but nonetheless it has often not been available or has not been publicized despite its usefulness." Patients clearly deserved to know which hospitals failed to meet safety standards. "Although 'shopping' for a hospital may not be in vogue," he wrote, "greater dissemination of information and wide public awareness might contribute to more hospital economy, especially if the public begins to question costs that appear to be out of line with what others are charging." Denenberg concluded, "the public may not be in a position to shop for a hospital, especially in view of a doctor's requirements and his hospital connections, but it is entitled to information that will permit comparisons."[21]

As of the early 1970s, the pressure that consumer advocates such as Denenberg could bring to bear in prying open existing data sources was still limited. Easily caricatured as "anti-business," Denenberg met with stiff resistance from the insurance industry. He left the commissioner's position in 1974 to run unsuccessfully for the U.S. Senate. Significantly, he found a second, rewarding career as a journalist and television personality in Philadelphia, where he pioneered a muckraking, "shame on you" style of reportage that has since become a staple of the American news industry. Whereas government officials providing consumer information faced charges of being "anti-business," television personalities could offer far more critical perspectives as a form of news provided by an independent press. So a combative style that did not work well in government service proved very successful with a viewing audience composed of discontented consumers, who agreed with his conviction that "the public has been screwed long enough," as Denenberg put it.[22]

From Shoppers' Guides to Hospital Report Cards

In the early 1970s, health care critics demanded more objective information on and greater institutional transparency in the health care system, requests that they presented as rational and social scientific in spirit. Yet as in the cases of the Prince George's County directory and the Philadelphia shoppers' guide to hospitals, their requests were highly politicized. The concept of a consumer buying guide to health care, as it first appeared in the 1970s, was a tool of political advocacy, championed by critics of the health care "establishment." But over the next two decades, profound changes in the health care system brought the concept of the educated health consumer from the periphery to the mainstream of policy thinking. This shift reflected a convergence of economic, political, and cultural trends, among them the steep rise in health care costs, the growing influence of economics on health policy discourse, the post-Watergate pressure for greater transparency in government, and the renewed emphasis on personal responsibility and accountability. These developments coincided with the rapid development of computer-assisted technologies that greatly facilitated data collection and analysis. All these trends converged to create what scholars term a new "era of accountability" in which information sources designed for the use of patients/consumers would flourish.[23]

The "era of accountability" reflected first and foremost the vast increase in federal investment in health care following the creation of Medicare and Medicaid in the mid-1960s. These new government programs generated massive databases concerning physicians and hospital practice, as well as creating intense pressures for cost containment. In addition, the federalization of medical care transformed the scope and significance of already established forms of assessment and accreditation. A case in point was the Joint Commission's program of hospital accreditation; hospitals now had to have the JCAH's stamp of approval in order to receive Medicare and Medicaid funding.

At the same time as federal agencies and accrediting bodies were compiling more such information, new computer-assisted information technologies emerged that were far more effective in processing it. As noted earlier, the kind of quality assessment done in earlier decades relied on relatively simple technologies, such as typewriters and carbon paper, and the first consumer buying guides produced by Nader's protégés were done on mimeograph machines. In other words, none of these early technologies of knowledge used complex systems of information retrieval and analysis. The rapid advance of both computer hardware and software eventually made possible a kind of quality assessment only dreamed of by reformers and bureaucrats prior to 1970.

The pathway from computers to consumer report cards was by no means a direct one. The first effect of the computer revolution was not to democratize information but rather to create a new group of experts; in the health care realm, that group was the health services researchers, whose studies, like those of Flexner and Codman, were not meant to inform individual patients' choices, but rather to influence policy makers and institutional leaders. But as we shall see, the birth of health services research eventually helped to create the kind of consumer-oriented data bases that Nader and Denenberg had in mind.

Starting in the 1970s, integrated circuits and miniaturization made possible a new generation of computers, including "supercomputers" capable of processing huge amounts of data, and minicomputers able to process smaller amounts of data for individual researchers and businesses. Moreover, these computers were increasingly being linked together into systems that allowed them to communicate with each other. With each passing year, electronic computers got smaller in size, larger in memory, faster in operation, and easier to operate.

Computer-assisted information technologies allowed for the collection, storage, retrieval, analysis, and communication of health data on a scale hitherto unimaginable. The great leap forward in electronic processing made it possible to do far more sophisticated forms of evaluation. The computer "revolution" facilitated the spread of a new kind of systems-oriented thinking that had originated in business and government circles during the late 1950s and 1960s. A case in point was Avedis Donabedian, a physician and public health professor at the University of Michigan. In his influential 1966 article, "Evaluating the Quality of Medical Care," which appeared in the *Milbank Memorial Fund Quarterly*, Donabedian proposed a system of evaluating structure, process, and outcome as a means to measure quality. Although Donabedian's approach did not require complex computations, much less the use of computers, it outlined a systems approach that was seemingly tailor made for electronic data collection and analysis.[24]

The convergence of systems thinking and computer-assisted technologies spurred the growth of health services research. In the 1970s and early 1980s, researchers began more rigorously to track the outcomes of medical intervention, from the number of particular procedures performed to the rate of hospital-based infections. As might be expected, these assessments uncovered many areas in which providers and hospitals were not performing either consistently or well.[25]

The work of Jack Wennberg at the Dartmouth Medical School was particularly influential in this regard. Like Donabedian, Wennberg was a physician with a strong background in epidemiology who became interested in the problem of local practice variations. Wennberg observed that despite their standardized training, physicians in different communities practiced medicine in highly variable ways that could not be explained by the characteristics of the communities' patient populations. Wennberg began to document local variations in medical practice, which he found to be extensive, and developed new methods of what he termed "outcomes research" to account for them. Like Codman's "end results system," Wennberg's analysis of practice variations did not require computer-assisted technologies, yet the growing ease of data gathering and manipulation made possible by the new generation of computers greatly enhanced the scope and legitimacy of such studies. It should be noted that the initial focus of Wennberg's work was not to identify and discipline individual physicians, but rather to document practice differences that should be addressed by the medical profession, through medical schools and medical societies.[26]

But here another development intervened to take health services research in a different direction. The concept of outcomes research resonated with another key development in the 1970s and early 1980s, namely the growth of the managed competition movement. As envisioned by economist Alan Enthoven and physician Paul Ellwood, managed competition would improve health care delivery by changing the economic incentives given to both provider and consumer. By linking payment systems to the pursuit of greater cost effectiveness and therapeutic efficacy, the American health care system could be dramatically improved. New forms of outcomes measurement and management were essential to this restructuring of health care economics; as Paul Ellwood explained in a 1997 article, outcomes research constituted a "technology of patient experience" that could be used to improve health care delivery. The managed competition movement became an important conduit through which the "informed patient, informed choice" formulation entered policy thinking.[27]

Early proponents of outcomes research had certainly envisioned their work as being useful to the patient/consumer. But their work was extremely abstruse, to say the least, and as such, primarily aimed at elite policy makers and not at end users. But the growing legitimacy of outcomes research, coupled with the managed competition philosophy, created a powerful impetus to develop new forms of rating and ranking that packed a more direct policy punch. Calls for public accountability resonated powerfully in a post-Watergate era, marked by the 1974 amendment of the Freedom of Information Act (FOIA, first passed in 1966) to make it much stronger. In this climate, it seemed only logical that institutional information sources be opened up and subjected to more critical analysis on patients' behalf. Even as other aspects of managed competition sparked enormous resistance, the concept of information disclosure as a service to consumers gained increasing appeal.

The first and most obvious target for this new spirit of disclosure was the Health Care Finance Administration (HCFA), the government body charged with overseeing the taxpayer-funded services delivered through Medicare and Medicaid. Soon after Medicare's founding in 1965, the HCFA began to set up a national network of "professional review organizations" (PROs) to monitor patient care. By 1973 its information database was substantial enough to attract the interest of Public Citizen's Health Research Group, which tried, through congressional petition and lawsuits, to have that data released to the public. Initially, those efforts were in vain; as Sidney Wolfe lamented to *Washington Post* reporter Victor Cohn, "we meet every kind of resistance you can imagine to the public's right to know." But with growing pressures for economic reform and consumer empowerment, the idea of publicly disclosing HCFA data gradually gained respectability. For example, in 1981, the prestigious Institute of Medicine endorsed the public disclosure of hospital mortality data to, in its words, "enhance consumer choice" and force medical institutions to have "public accountability."[28]

In 1986, Secretary of Health and Human Services Otis Bowen appointed William Roper, described in the *Washington Post* as "a public health officer with a strong belief in medical accountability," as the HCFA's head. Both Roper and his boss were political conservatives as well as physicians, so the idea of accountability appealed to them. When Roper suggested to his staff that hospital mortality rates become part of the PRO review, they were reluctant. Still, as he later explained, he decided "this was something I wanted to do, not because it's legislatively required but because it's right." Roper went ahead and ordered his staff to prepare a preliminary study of 142 hospitals. Initially, it should be noted, he did not intend to make this report public, believing that the data would be too difficult for the average American to interpret. But the *New York Times* heard of the study and announced its intention to sue for its release under the Freedom of Information Act. At the advice of the HCFA's counsel, Roper then released the report in December 1987.[29]

The report received extensive coverage in the news media, with particular emphasis on the local hospitals that got bad "grades" from the HCFA. Observers immediately pointed out the many flaws of the data, flaws that had made HCFA officials reluctant to release the data in the first place. For example, the data analysis could not sufficiently correct for how seriously ill a hospital's patients were; the sicker the patients, the more likely they were to die, and thus to inflate the institution's mortality rates. Yet for all the reservations, the data release was hailed as a "revolutionary first step in giving consumers an objective measure of the quality of care in individual hospitals," as the *Washington Post* reported. As Jack Christy of the American Association of Retired Person's Public Policy Institute told Victor Cohn of the *Post*, "We've finally cracked the reticence, the guild protective mentality" that had denied the public such useful information.[30]

The HCFA's 1987 release of hospital mortality data exemplifies a pattern that would recur repeatedly over the next two decades. By taking advantage of new standards of public accountability, patient advocacy groups and health care policy reformers found far greater support for opening up institutional databases than had earlier generations of health care critics. With the assistance of newspaper journalists eager and willing to file FOIA requests, the barriers against data release began to weaken. Yet with growing disclosure of information came a predictable cycle of criticism: the data was incomplete and difficult to interpret, leading to redoubled efforts to refine data collection. This pattern, apparent with earlier grading exercises, including the Flexner report and the early guinea pig books, would be repeated over and over again: the data was made available and then immediately criticized for not being good enough, misleading, or hard to use. These criticisms only reinforce the assumption that if only better information could be compiled and distilled into forms that consumers could use, the information Rx would have the desired policy results. Hence the cycle would begin again.

Consumer Information as Marketing Device

But the quest for more objective and rational use of public databases failed to take into account another powerful trend of the 1970s and 1980s, namely the parallel rise of market research and health care advertising. At the same time as patient advocacy groups and health policy reformers were pressing for greater consumer access to information, important players in the health care arena sought to legitimate another kind of consumer "information," namely better marketing and advertising methods. The same economic and cultural factors that led to the growing demand for public accountability also brought about a higher tolerance for marketing and advertising of health care products and services. The rapid commercialization of the report card concept highlights a critical feature of the American policy environment: the rise of health services *research*, in the spirit of Donabedian and Wennberg, was accompanied by the equally, if not more robust growth of health services *marketing*.

Although marketing and advertising were by no means new to American health care, their penetration of the field had been constrained by the resistance of the medical profession and the hospital industry. Until the 1970s, the kind of commercial suasions used to promote automobiles or appliances were viewed as unseemly when applied to the public's choice of a doctor or a hospital. But, ironically, given the hostility that both consumer groups and health service researchers had long expressed toward the advertising industry, their championing of consumer information helped to facilitate the widening scope of health care advertising and marketing efforts.

As early as 1971, the same year Herb Denenberg published his first "buyer's guide," two business school professors, Gerald Zaltman and Ilan Vertinksy, published an influential article in the *Journal of Marketing* outlining the promising future of health care marketing. As they explained, the emphasis on consumer choice had the potential to help business interests breach longstanding barriers to commercial health care promotion. As public and private health care policy makers began to experiment with more market-oriented approaches to health care, they invested more in marketing and advertising as forms of consumer information as well. And like their counterparts in health services research, marketing professionals appreciated the ways that new computer-assisted technologies could improve the quality and scope of their research.[31]

The much publicized entry in the 1980s of private for-profit hospital chains accelerated this competitive ethos among American hospitals. For-profit chains such as Humana and Hospital Corporation of America invested heavily in marketing, forcing the nonprofit hospitals to respond in kind. Starting in the late 1970s, a host of new marketing firms moved into the health care field, offering their expertise to hospitals trying to survive the "marketization" of health care. Over the course of the 1980s, hospital expenditures on marketing and advertising grew rapidly.[32]

The published proceedings of the Academy of Health Care Marketing, a division of the American Marketing Association, reveal how enthusiastically the marketing field adopted the information Rx. A good example was the 1989 presentation to the academy by Robert Kimmel, the vice president for marketing and communications for Albert Einstein Medical Center in Philadelphia. He began by describing the events of the past decade as "the story . . . of the epic struggle to decide who controls our medical information," and the "incredible power that comes from controlling that information." Until very recently, he noted, doctors had exercised virtually total control over what patients knew, a "traditional model of medical information" that he characterized as "about as useful as a buggy whip in a Mercedes." Today's public, Kimmel included, had come to realize what doctors did not, that the key to better health care lay in effective sharing of information. But "in our society, it's easier to make an informed choice about microwave ovens than about doctors," and as a result, "the public is dazed and confused, bombarded with questions they can't answer *because they don't have the right information*" [emphasis in original].[33]

As Kimmel's speech went on to make clear, the kind of information he had in mind differed dramatically from that envisioned by his contemporaries Sidney Wolfe or Jack Wennberg. His "information revolution" consisted of better executed advertising and marketing campaigns. As he concluded, "It's the job of marketers—the professional communicators—to provide the information as effectively as possible." But that information should be designed as a means to promote one's own institution, in his case Einstein Medical Center. Tellingly, the title of his talk was "How to Be Ethical While Eating Your Competitor's Lunch."[34]

For hospital marketing experts, consumer-oriented appeals figured centrally in strategies to break the physician monopoly on referrals. As their research revealed, most patients followed their physician's recommendation in choosing a hospital. Thus in order to succeed, hospital marketing efforts had to disrupt that traditional pattern of referral, either by influencing patients to pressure their physicians to use a particular hospital, or by getting patients to choose the hospital first, and then find a physician affiliated with it.[35]

As part of this effort, marketing firms began to work with hospitals to present the growing volume of outcomes data in the most attractive light. They also began to conduct their own marketing surveys to help buff the institution's public image. As marketing firms realized, the "era of accountability" posed some potential dangers to their hospital clients. In a paper presented at the 1988 academy meeting, titled "Data Driven Quality Differentiation: Using PRO Mortality Data to Market your Hospital," the authors, both researchers with advanced marketing degrees, reviewed the PRO/HCFA developments to acquaint their audience with both its risks and benefits. They emphasized that mortality data needed to be used "professionally, ethically, and properly," in order not to heighten consumer distrust of medical institutions, which they admitted was already high. Given that "the health care industry is already distrusted and reeling under attack from consumer groups, employers and Congress," outcomes data should be used carefully "to avoid the scenario of hospitals racing against each other, on a muddy track, in an endless mortality data derby where nobody can emerge as a winner." To prevent that from happening, they suggested more "subtle" use of such data: negative outcomes could be used internally to encourage improvement, while positive data should be emphasized in public statements and marketing efforts.[36]

News You Can Use

Neither of the new forms of accountability that emerged in the 1980s—the massive data dumps from the HCFA nor the hospital marketing campaigns endorsed by the "other" AMA—met the demand for reliable, usable information for the health care consumer. Thus, into an already confused information marketplace, there emerged yet another contender for the role of the "honest broker," namely the mass media. The trendsetter in this regard was *U.S. News and World Report*, which began in 1990 to publish a special consumers' guide to hospitals. The hospital issue copied the formula *U.S. News* had developed during the 1980s to produce college and law school rankings. By distilling evidence of an institution's reputation into an easily comprehensible rating system, the magazine offered its readers "news you can use," as the editors christened it.

The first *U.S. News and World Report* hospital issue explained why the news magazine decided to enter the business of providing consumer ratings for hospitals. As the authors noted, although hospitals were "prodigious data generators," yet with the exception of the HCFA's mortality rates, a data set of debatable value, none of it was in a form truly usable by consumers. "Since no medical authority—or anyone else—had ever devised yardsticks for rating hospitals that are both useful and statistically valid, *U.S. News* had to create its own." Realizing that hospitals varied enormously across departments, the magazine staff decided to focus on twelve different specialties, "from AIDS to urology."[37]

To develop the ratings, the *U.S. News* staff sent a confidential survey form to almost fifteen hundred physicians in those specialties, asking them to list the top ten hospitals in their area. It was in essence a poll of experts meant to be shared with the public. It should be noted that their method here differed from the law school rankings, in that the staff did not seek to develop a rigid numerical ranking but only a list of "the best" institutions in no hierarchical order. The survey results were used to winnow the 6,500 hospitals in the United States down to a list of the best 57. As the authors of the list emphasized, the results "should not imply that other hospitals cannot deliver excellent care," or that the hospitals appearing on the list were always perfect. But the *U.S. News* staff felt that their list represented an excellent starting point.[38]

Moreover, in addition to the list itself, the magazine offered useful advice about how to assess the markers of quality care. For example, the first report suggested that "people who need surgery should ask a surgeon about volume" of procedures done and noted that new treatments for kidney stones required a hospital to have a "lithotripter, an expensive machine that hammers the stone with ultrasonic blows." Subsequent reports continued in the same tradition. For example, in 1991, the report included a review of the year's developments in consumer health information, from the Joint Commission on Accreditation of Healthcare Organization's plans to measure the quality of medical specialties, to Blue Cross/Blue Shield's decision to steer patients to selected organ transplant centers. The same issue reported on the Health Care Financing Administration's efforts to develop more sophisticated versions of its hospital mortality data and described the growing efforts on the part of state governments to equip consumers with better decision-making tools.[39]

Having found a winning formula, U.S. News stuck with it, and has continued to publish the hospital ratings issue ever since. This feature effectively combined the solidity of numbers—survey results and ratings—with suggestions about quality indicators to look for and questions to ask. In effect, the magazine positioned itself as an honest broker of information upon which readers could depend. As the staff continued to maintain, "despite the growing information from both sides of the hospital bed on the quality of care, the U.S. News survey is the only broad assessment available." U.S. News's hospital rankings came to constitute news themselves: each year, local newspapers reported which of the area's hospitals made it into the news magazine's ratings.[40]

"Best hospital" lists soon gave rise to comparable "best doctors" lists, created in similar ways: large numbers of doctors were asked to name the best specialists in their community, and the resulting names distilled to short lists of the individuals most frequently named by their peers. For example, by the early 1990s, two companies competed for the market in guides to New York City's "top doctors," one developed by a computer software analyst named Richard Topp, the other by a physician named John Connolly. Of the two, the latter proved more successful, in part because of its agreement as of 1997 to let New York Magazine publish an abridged version of its best doctors list; this feature has remained a regular offering of the magazine ever since. Similarly, other city magazines made an annual "top doctors" issue a staple of their publication strategy. In a 1999 article about such magazines, Jim Dowden, director of the City and Regional Magazine Association, described "such city mag chestnuts as top restaurants, top doctors, and best buys" as the issues that kept those publications in business. As he put it, "it's the service journalism, not the hot model that really sells."[41] City mags bare it, and grin.

Not surprisingly, the disclosure of information about "bad" doctors proved to be more difficult than publicizing lists of "good" doctors. Starting in the 1970s, both the American Medical Association and many state medical boards had developed master files of problematic physicians, but they did not share the contents with anyone, even the profession's own credentialing bodies. Thus doctors convicted of malpractice who lost their medical licenses in one state could simply move to another and resume practicing. As the number of medical malpractice suits rose in the 1970s and 1980s, raising concerns about a malpractice "epidemic," this reticence came under increasing criticism.

At a time when they agreed on little else, conservatives and liberals found common cause in cracking down on "bad" doctors. Thus in 1986, the U.S. Congress passed the Health Care Quality Improvement Act, which provided for the creation of a National Practitioner Data Bank (NPDB). The new law required that malpractice insurance companies, state licensing boards, and other organizations report cases of negligence and incompetence to the data bank.[42]

During the hearings about the 1986 law, consumer advocacy groups, chief among them the Public Citizen's Health Research Group, argued that the new database should be open to the public, while the AMA and other medical groups argued just as fiercely that its use should be restricted. In the end, the bill creating the National Practitioner Data Bank (NPDB) exempted it from the terms of the Freedom of Information Act and limited its use to hospitals, state licensing authorities, and professional societies. Public Citizen's Health Research Group immediately lodged a court challenge to that limitation, but the courts have consistently ruled in favor of physicians' right to privacy as opposed to the public's right to know. But in the process, Public Citizen secured itself access to the data bank, as well as a seat on the NPDB's governing board. Using that access, the group created its own bad doctor list, which it publishes as a service to consumers.[43]

Recent Developments and Critical Reflections

As this brief overview suggests, by the advent of the Internet in the mid-1990s, the consumer information Rx was already well established as both a policy goal and a set of practices. Since the 1990s, the intersection of trends toward consumer empowerment and powerful new computational capacities has resulted in a remarkable democratization of health information. As a result, today's patient consumers now have access to a dizzying array of information sources. But what was true in the 1970s remains true today: what consumer activists, health services researchers, market researchers, and journalists mean by the invocation of the "godword" of information is highly variable and at times contradictory.

The growing demand for economic discipline, efficiency, cost control, and quality improvement has played a key role in the creation of new information sources. From an initial focus on hospital mortality rates, health researchers' efforts have broadened to include other markers of quality care. In 1993, the National Committee on Health Care Quality introduced its first Healthcare Effectiveness Data and Information Set (HEDIS), including a much wider array of measures designed to help consumers choose among health plans. Subsequent versions of the HEDIS data have expanded to include measures of patient satisfaction. In 1995, the Centers for Medicare and Medicaid Services introduced its own Health Consumer Assessment of Health Care Providers and Systems, or HCAHPS, to do a better job of capturing patients' views of their experiences. Meanwhile, a new generation of expert groups hoping to function as "honest brokers" of these databases has emerged, among them the 1990 National Committee for Quality Assurance, the 1997 Advisory Commission on Consumer Protection and Quality in the Health Care Industry, and the Institute of Medicine's Committee on Quality of Health Care in America. These national trends have been paralleled by similar developments at the state level. Since so much of health care delivery occurs in the context of local government, states have developed their own consumer health information initiatives.[44]

Commercial forms of consumer information, in the form of sophisticated hospital marketing campaigns and magazine guides to the best hospitals, have also continued to flourish. The consumer guide concept pioneered by *U.S. News and World Report* almost twenty years ago continues to find new expressions. The peer-to-peer evaluation method initially used with physician opinion leaders is now being used with consumers as well, as evident in the entrance of Zagat and other companies into the doctor rating business. As mentioned in the introduction, the Zagat-WellPoint collaboration is but the latest example of this phenomenon. Building on the success of similar surveys devoted to ranking university professors, the doctor-rating Web sites have expanded very quickly. WellPoint's decision to collaborate with Zagat testifies to the growing popularity of this kind of information source; a major player in the health insurance industry, WellPoint is the owner of Blue Cross of California and the second largest health insurer in the country, covering one in nine Americans.[45]

Yet this deluge of consumer oriented information has not necessarily produced the results promised by its advocates. In the first place, it is an approach to health care choice rooted in the needs of affluent Americans with the financial and educational resources required to "shop" for health care. The principles of consumer driven health care are not designed for low income Americans with no health insurance and limited literacy. As critics have long complained, this kind of consumer-driven health care simply perpetuates the inequitable thrust of the American health care system. Yet even the target audience of middle-class educated consumers finds many of the new consumer information sources hard to use. Many studies have attested to the fact that consumers find the rankings and ratings produced by competing groups both difficult to access and hard to understand.

For example, a 2000 survey of consumers done by the Kaiser Family Foundation and the Agency for Healthcare Research Quality found that fewer than 10 percent of those surveyed made use of the comparative quality ratings provided by government agencies, employers, consumer groups, or the media. The vast majority—70 percent—continue to rely on personal recommendations from family and friends when it comes to picking a physician, a hospital, or a health plan. More recent roll-outs of allegedly consumer-oriented databases suggest that they still have far to go in becoming user friendly even for their target audience of the literate and concerned patient. When the federal government released its first comprehensive results from the HCAHPS patient satisfaction surveys, even health care experts commented that the new information was not easy to use. As one nurse executive put it, "There's a lot to maneuver; I think it's going to take the average consumer a little while" to understand it.[46] Patient/consumers also know that quality measures do not necessarily include the kind of issues that concern them. Readers' criticisms of *New York Magazine*'s "best doctors" issue are a case in point. In a recent year, one man wrote in to complain that the magazine's "boosterish approach" promoted a "celebrity" doctor system, and failed to ask what was for many consumers a "critical question," namely, did the doctor accept health insurance? The reader reported his own experience of consulting one of the listed physicians about performing a life-saving operation for his son, only to find out the doctor did not accept health insurance. Other readers complained that the issue neglected specialties such as podiatry and naturopathy. As one wrote, "Your paean to the medical industry perpetuates the myth that alternative doctors are unqualified and not to be trusted when it comes to serious disease."[47]

From a policy makers' standpoint, perhaps the most serious criticism of rankings and ratings aimed at consumers is their unintended impact on provider and institutional behavior. In theory, institutions and individuals are supposed to use performance measures as a goad to do better; for example, public reporting of hospitals' rates of serious infection or providers' rates of success with a particular procedure will create a positive pressure for them to improve in those areas. To be sure, some studies suggest that public reporting is indeed having that desirable effect. For example, Wisconsin's efforts to standardize and improve quality in its hospitals have produced encouraging results.[48]

But in practice, ratings and rankings also function to "judge and control," in the words of Wendy Espeland and Michael Sauder, and thus encourage "the proliferation of gaming strategies." As they have shown in their study of law school rankings, awareness of being monitored leads subjects to alter their behavior in unexpected ways. Instead of concentrating on improving legal education, schools figure out ways to "game" the system so that their rankings improve. They note there is no reason to think this phenomenon is limited to law schools. As more health care institutions have be brought into what Espeland and Sauder refer to as the modern "audit culture" and "culture of accountability," the trend toward gaming has likely increased.[49]

A troubling example of this phenomenon was reported in the *Annals of Internal Medicine* in 2005. Researchers reported that since New York had begun publicly to report on physicians' performance, almost 80 percent of cardiologists surveyed reported that they avoided treating critically ill patients because they feared a bad outcome would affect their report cards. Likewise, a more comprehensive review by Rachel Werner and David A. Asch published that same year in the *Journal of the American Medical Association* warned of the same problem. While expressing agreement with the goals of quality improvement, they concluded that "the value of publicly reporting quality information is largely undemonstrated" and may have "unintended and negative consequences on health care."[50]

Predictably, then, given the highly competitive nature both of health care provision and mass media, the proliferation of report cards, ratings, and rankings has itself become a source of consumer confusion. Consumers now require guides to the guides: for example, the Medical Library Association's consumer health section now provides its own "top 100 list" of "health websites you can trust" in order to help consumers distinguish between "good" and 'bad" information sources. Its list of criteria testifies to just how complicated this process has become; Web sites are judged by "credibility, sponsorship/authorship, content, audience, currency, disclosure, purpose, links, design, interactivity, and caveats" In order to be well informed, consumers now have to devote even more time to verifying the source and credibility of the many information sources being offered them. Again, this is a style of information seeking and use deeply biased against Americans with limited income and time.[51]

If history is any guide, the cycle of more consumer information sources, followed by more questions and criticisms, will continue unabated in the future. Many different groups will continue to vie for primacy as the consumers' trusted guide to health care information. Marketing firms will continue to spin quality information into advertising plans that benefit their clients. Health care institutions and providers will continue to game the ratings system to try to improve their "report cards." Last but not least, patient-consumers will continue to bypass formal ratings and rankings to follow their "gut," as Sanjay Gupta recommended in an article on the 2008 Zagat/Wellpoint venture. As he noted, "it's hard to imagine Dr. Gregory House, the famously cranky lead character of the eponymous TV show, scoring very high on that burgundy scale, but he's an awfully smart doc all the same."[52]

As this historical overview suggests, better information sources for health consumers have not turned out to be a "magic bullet" capable of correcting the dysfunctionality of the American health care system. The limitations of the consumer information Rx reflect the fact that the consumer information revolution has been inseparable from the broader "marketization" of health that has occurred over the last fifty years. Information itself has become a commodity produced and circulated by many different actors. The "godword" of information has come to have many different, sometimes contradictory meanings: as a neutral set of data, an economic driver of choice, a "right" of the modern consumer, and a sophisticated means of business competition. The end result is a complicated, chaotic, potentially toxic information environment, far from the world of rational decision making envisioned by the early champions of a more rational process of consumer choice.

Starting in the 1970s, consumer advocates effectively used market-oriented arguments that patients needed better information to make better choices to challenge the expert monopoly on information. As demands for accountability and transparency accelerated in the 1980s and 1990s, the report card and its many variants emerged as versatile tools that consumers could use to improve their satisfaction with health care choices, while also exercising a positive discipline on a decentralized health care system.

But, ironically, the growing marketization of health care diluted the impact of rigorous analysis by encouraging the growth of more sophisticated marketing and advertising strategies. Faced with stiff competition, hospitals, marketing firms, and news outlets all adapted consumer-oriented information guides such as report cards and ratings to promote their own institutional and economic interests. As a consequence, consumers have been bombarded with a deluge of health related advertising, and the difference between advertising and information has become increasingly difficult to define. Consumers now need a report card to help them choose their information sources.

Thus the hospital executive's image of the "dazed and confused consumer" circa 1989 still seems quite apt today. What sounds good in theory—better information leads to better choices—has proven extremely difficult in practice. While it has been productive of much good, the consumer health information "revolution" has not resulted in a markedly more efficient health care system. Not the least of the reasons for this failure is the fact that American health care is delivered within a highly competitive, market-oriented culture in which information is simply a synonym for advertising.

Yet we do not want to throw out the baby with the bathwater: as Arnold M. Epstein, the physician who heads Harvard's department of health care policy and management, points out. Even if patients find the new quality report cards hard to use, "shedding sunlight on medical practice is unquestionably health medicine for patients." While flawed in many ways, the consumer health revolution has become a policy fact of life in the United States. There is no returning to the pre-1970s era in which information and accountability did not figure as goals of policy making. Rather the key to a better future lies in having a more realistic understanding of what informed consumers can and cannot accomplish.[53]

When New Is Old

Professional Medical Liability in the Information Age

One of the more common refrains about health information technology (HIT) is its potential to heighten professional liability exposure as a result of privacy infringement, security leaks, or misuse of an emerging technology.[1] The introduction of a new technology can elevate risk of liability as a result of both anticipated and unforeseen consequences flowing from its use. But where health care is concerned, society increasingly is coming to expect that technology breakthroughs will mean better access to more and better information to assist medical decision making. This heightened expectation involves more than just consumer-initiated online Web searches or aggregated patient data regarding performance at the health system level (e.g., hospital comparison report cards). The traditional physician/patient relationship largely rests on a paternalistic information asymmetry. In that asymmetrical relationship, physicians hold superior knowledge that they mete out, as appropriate, to patients.

To a certain extent, technology-enabled information will likely intensify the expectation that physicians will be on top of the very latest studies and data regarding what will work for a patient's ailment, as well as the relative strengths, limitations (and possibly the costs) of various treatment approaches. Patients also expect that their physicians will discuss these options with them as part of their course of treatment. The information technology that undergirds this growing set of expectations should begin to spread more rapidly as a result of 2009 federal legislation that formally makes information technology-enabled health care a matter of national public policy through the establishment of a system of rewards and penalties for physician and hospital adoption.[2]

Technology-enabled health information can elevate certain liability risks, but the converse is equally important. Indeed, as HIT adoption becomes more common, a physician's lack of HIT capability may itself be a cause of liability. In the medical negligence context, the law historically has pushed physicians toward using information. As the health care system moves toward technology-enabled information, these longstanding legal principles serve as a reminder that significant legal risks arise when health professionals ignore available information, conceal or withhold information, or fail to seek and make active use of reasonably accessible information. This link between health care and health information means that as the information context for medical practice evolves, so will the legal risks associated with failing to practice health care without using modern health information practice tools.

HIT adoption among U.S. physicians is still relatively limited; indeed, the best evidence suggests that as of 2008, only 17 percent of physicians used electronic health records in office settings and only 4 percent possessed what might be considered by experts to be a fully functional electronic health record.[3] But as with other fundamental advances in health care, HIT ultimately will become sufficiently widespread so that professional norms will swing toward its use, and at this point, the liabilities associated with the failure to use technology will begin to emerge.

This chapter begins with a brief overview of the longstanding relationship between medical professionalism and health information and also considers the core elements of HIT and the ways in which HIT may change the ways in which medical professionals acquire, use and impart health information to patients. The chapter then examines various legal theories that long predate the introduction of HIT but reflect the extent to which expectations about professionalism and information traditionally have shaped concepts of liability. The chapter concludes with a discussion of how these longstanding theories might emerge in a technology-enabled information age and the possible ways in which medical liability reforms ultimately might be used to spur HIT adoption among physicians.

Overview

Medical Practice, Health Care Information, and Professional Negligence

The heart of medical professionalism can be found in the degree of knowledge and expertise that elevates the medical and health care professions above other potential sources of health care and shapes the special relationship between professionals and patients. The knowledge and information platform on which medical practice rests in turn gives rise to specific types of theories of professional negligence. The starting point for understanding this link between knowledge and information on the one hand and liability on the other is a more general overview of medical negligence theory.

As with any vast endeavor operating within a complex legal environment, the health care enterprise raises an array of legal issues ranging from professional and corporate medical negligence to liability under various regulatory and financial laws. Indeed, health care professionals seem to be in a constant state of legal exposure, a far cry from the more exalted position they once held under the law.[4] It is fair to say that the past several decades have witnessed the expansion of professional and corporate medical liability even as the law has come to shield insurers and health plan administrators from the consequences of negligence in connection with the administration of coverage plans.[5] It is also fair to say that among all forms of medical liability, medical malpractice litigation raises the deepest passions within the profession, because it strikes at the heart of the physician-patient relationship itself.

The legal principles that shape the law of medical negligence are highly patient-centered. That is, the theory of medical liability grows out of the relationship of trust between a specific physician and a specific patient,[6] and the concept of medical liability is shaped by the duties that physicians owe to individual patients as opposed to those owed to society at large.

In medical negligence cases, a physician's legal liability is measured against the professional standard of care,[7] a concept that is established through the presentation of admissible evidence that demonstrates both the appropriate standard of conduct in a particular case, as well as the degree to which a defendant's conduct may have fallen below the particular professional standard involved. As with medical practice itself, the professional standard of care is both evolving and dynamic and is influenced by advances in science, technology, society, and culture.[8]

Under older common law principles, the professional standard of care actually shielded physicians from liability, since liability was measured in terms of the particular customs of the profession, as testified to by professionals from the same or a similar locality.[9] Under modern principles, embodied in the laws of most states (health care liability concepts are grounded in the common law and statutes that codify or alter common law principles),[10] liability tends to rest on a more objective, evidence-based concept of "reasonable prudence." Under this framework, the custom of the profession has only limited relevance; more important is what is considered *reasonable* in view of objective standards of training and knowledge. Especially in the case of the medical specialties, the concept of reasonableness is attuned to national expectations and standards rather than local practice (although actual local practice conditions become relevant when determining if liability should be found). Thus, for example, an expert from Boston is considered qualified to testify in a medical negligence case involving health care in Washington, D.C., because the expectations of Washington D.C. physicians are shaped by national standards. This concept of a professional standard of care that rests on national norms carries important implications for negligence allegations in connection with the use of technology.[11]

The question of liability frequently turns on information: what information a physician might have had about a patient's condition; whether the physician acted with sufficient knowledge of treatment alternatives and their risks; or how the physician used information in treating and counseling a patient. Indeed, it is fair to say that the ability to secure and translate information into appropriate knowledge and action is a fundamental aspect of medical professionalism; as a result, liability cases often rest on allegations that somehow a health professional failed to acquire, use, and disclose information properly about treatments and management of conditions.

Even a cursory reading of leading cases shows that, like professionalism itself, negligence in relation to health information lies at the heart of much malpractice litigation. Many of the most common types of negligence claims in some way rest on information: the failure to appropriately use reasonable available information when diagnosing or treating a patient; the failure to use information regarding the management of a particular condition, thereby depriving the patient of a chance of recovery; the failure to adopt technology innovations that would both provide a safer work environment while also improving knowledge regarding the patient's health status and reaction to a course of treatment; the failure to convey adequate information to a patient regarding the material risks and benefits associated with various treatment options; and the withholding or concealing of information about medical errors and poor quality, thereby heightening risks to patient health and safety.

Health Information Technology

Health information technology introduces a new dimension to any discussion of the professional standard of care and the resulting risk of medical negligence if conduct falls below the standard. HIT has the potential to increase exponentially the amount, range, and quality of useful and relevant information available to a treating or consulting physician. HIT also increases a physician's ability to translate knowledge into higher quality patient care with more limited potential for error. This potential for health information to translate into better care can be seen in both the clinical care enterprise through which patients move as well as in the level of information that patients receive as they undergo diagnosis and treatment. In sum, by facilitating the acquisition and use of current and high quality information, HIT can be expected ultimately to affect both questions of clinical quality and matters of health care transparency available to patients regarding their conditions, their treatments, and the cost of care.

In their report on the use of information technology in medicine, David Blumenthal and John Glaser note that a central question of the technology is "whether HIT is best viewed as one more in the long list of technologies" introduced into medical care "without great disruption" or whether the technology is "potentially transformative" in relation to the practice of medicine itself.[12] The answer to this question lies in a more exact understanding of what HIT is and its potential to alter fundamentally health care practice and social expectations about health care and health care professionals.

Blumenthal and Glaser note that HIT is actually a catch-all phrase for an "enormously diverse set of technologies"[13] that relate to information about patients and the process of care. Within this range of technologies the authors identify three—the electronic health record (EHR), the personal health record (PHR), and the clinical data exchange—as the most relevant to daily practice, and thus for the purposes of this chapter, the professional standard of care.

An EHR is defined in federal law as "a repository of consumer health status information in computer processable form used for clinical diagnosis and treatment for a broad array of clinical conditions."[14] In practical terms, the EHR encompasses a series of eight functionalities, four of which are considered "core" functions (health information and data, results management, order entry and support, and decision support).[15] These core functionalities allow the collection and storage of a broad array of patient data, computerized physician order entry, and computerized decision support regarding the care of specific patients. In effect, the technology makes an enormous amount of information about patients and treatments virtually immediately accessible to physicians.

PHRs are the logical result of the Health Insurance Portability and Accountability Act (HIPAA) Privacy Rule, which requires entities covered by the law to permit patients access to their medical records;[16] PHR technology is still evolving. Blumenthal and Glaser note that as of 2007, a PHR is most importantly a patient portal into his or her EHR, a means of viewing information that previously may not have been either known or accessible. As it evolves, the PHR can be expected to produce not only greater patient access to health information but also the opportunity for more frequent and probing levels of patient interaction with health professionals. Patients will be able to view and update information in their record, seek referrals, exchange information with physicians outside of a scheduled office visit, and in general be more actively engaged in their own health care management. Patients also will be more likely, using these portals, to be able to conduct online searches for information comparing the cost and quality of their health care. Over time, patients' expectations about what they know and when they know it will rise. In sum, even though medical records themselves may be owned by physicians (who in turn have a fiduciary duty to maintain and protect them on their patients' behalf), issues of ownership will become increasingly less relevant as a result of increasingly available PHR technology.[17]

Other aspects of EHR technology are also important, in particular the order entry support function, which permits greater speed and accuracy in connection with the transmission of diagnostic and treatment orders, and the decision support function, which offers physicians an effective bedside informational tool that can aid complex diagnostic and treatment decision-making. EHRs also will play a central role in the generation and submission of reports regarding health care quality and performance.

As of 2009, clinical data exchanges through centralized entities known as regional health information systems (RHIOs)[18] were evolving slowly. Part of the reason for this slowness is cost and the technological complexity of RHIOs;[19] part may be fundamental resistance to interoperability on the part of a health care industry focused on maintaining a competitive edge.[20]

Evidence regarding the effects of HIT on quality and safety is limited and contradictory. Research has shown that HIT can improve the quality of care; at the same time, however, the only rigorous studies to date have been conducted within controlled health care environments involving pioneering institutions that developed technology capabilities over a long time period. One prominent study has shown that EHR use in the current clinical and incentive environment does not necessarily lead to improvements in ambulatory care.[21] At least one study has shown that the process of adoption itself can actually lead to a spike in mortality.[22]

Bumpy results and complexity in adoption undoubtedly contribute to slow HIT diffusion rates in the United States, although as noted, the rate of diffusion has increased in recent years, particularly in ambulatory care settings.[23] Factors that may help explain the slowness of HIT adoption are its substantial initial and ongoing costs and the long absence of meaningful national policies aimed at achieving system-wide adoption.[24] This final

consideration—the lack of a clear national policy favoring adoption of HIT—
has been dramatically altered by the 2009 federal legislation to finance and
enable adoption and a "meaningful use" of technology. This decisive shift
toward a national policy of adoption can in turn be expected to fundamentally
alter over time the practice environment through which the professional standard of care is viewed. This transformation of medical care is occurring simultaneously with other types of movement, as the federal government applies
greater pressure on federal agencies to make information available to purchasers and consumers[25] and as legal barriers to the disclosure of health care
and pricing information fall.[26]

Another explanation for the slow rate of adoption may be actual and perceived legal barriers that inhibit adoption (such as concerns over greater liability for privacy and security breaches). There is also a natural tendency to resist
undertaking a technology improvement that can upend daily practice, at least
for a period of time. Even more fundamentally, physicians' opposition to the
adoption of HIT may spring from deeply held concerns about the degree to
which information technology will enable payers, regulators, and patients to
peer inside the black box of health care practice. HIT is not simply adding a
new gadget; it is a technology that can augment practice skills and tools while
at the same time revealing the inner workings of health care. And it is an expensive technology. The upfront investment and the ongoing maintenance costs
are high, and the practical potential for a return on investment, is low at least
from the perspective of any single medical group starting down the HIT road.

In a legal context, one interesting benefit of HIT adoption may be the extent
to which the type of clinical integration that technology can create across a
group of otherwise independent physicians may allow physicians to engage in
collective negotiation practices with insurers that otherwise would be prohib-
ited under federal antitrust law. This potential for technology-enabled clinical
integration to protect what otherwise would be an anticompetitive restraint
on trade was underscored by a 2007 advisory ruling from the Federal Trade
Commission (FTC) that allowed collective negotiations by a large medical
group operating under a unified governance structure and enabled through
HIT.[27] Even though the group was not operating at financial risk (an operating
arrangement that is required under FTC standards in order to qualify for a clear
antitrust law "safety zone"), the FTC nonetheless blessed the arrangement,
finding that physicians who would otherwise be competing were operating
under a common set of principles and had integrated their disparate practices
through the use of information technology. The technology used represented a
sizable financial investment for practice members: an initial contribution of

$7,000 per physician, additional hardware investments of $6,000–$7,000 per office, a $70 per month Internet connection fee, an initial loss of $3,200 in patient revenue to attend mandatory training in the use of HIT, and ongoing losses as a result of time spent in using the new system. These considerations were critical, because they showed a significant financial investment in the creation of an improved health care product, and a clearly integrated approach to health care. This willingness to clinically integrate ultimately was sufficient to overcome the FTC's concerns about the absence of competition in order to allow unified negotiating conduct that held the promise of improvements in the quality of care. Indeed, cases such as this one suggest that medicine ultimately may find a strong business case for HIT investment.

But even without a business case as an economic spur, the national policy movement toward establishing HIT as the operating norm for physicians will begin to alter the social and practice environment from which legal expectations of health care quality flow. It is true that as of 2007, as noted, less than 20 percent of physicians used a basic set of EHR functions in ambulatory practice in the United States, and only 4 percent used EHRs in their full functionalities.[28] These numbers can be expected to rise as the 2009 legislation takes hold and physicians and hospitals begin to respond to the reward and penalty system it creates.

The Professional Standard of Care
in the Context of Health Information

At its core, professionalism involves the use of information to aid the exercise of judgment by physicians on behalf of patients.[29] Because the core of medicine is about making treatment decisions,[30] both the common law and statutory law recognize a range of professional duties related to the acquisition, use, maintenance, and disclosure of information that creates the knowledge base on which medical practice rests. Because the professional duty of care incorporates duties related to health information, there are correspondingly a variety of ways in which a health professional can be held liable for information-related negligence.

The law recognizes several distinct classes of information-related duties for the medical profession: the general duty to furnish care and treatment in accordance with reasonable professional standards; the duty to use reasonable standards in creating, maintaining, and safeguarding patient information in medical records; and the duty of transparency. The duty of transparency encompasses the duty to disclose risks of treatment and to warn patients (and in certain circumstances, third parties) about material risks associated with health and health care, the duty to obtain informed patient consent to treatment, and the duty to disclose actual and potential conflicts of interest.

Adherence to the Professional Standard of Care

The obligation to practice in a manner consistent with the professional standard of care represents the bedrock principle upon which professional liability law rests. It is a duty that rests on centuries-old principles of common law, many of which have been expanded upon and modified by state statutes.[31] Some states continue to use professional liability standards that rely heavily on local custom when ascertaining both the standard of care and its breach;[32] other states may stress conformance with a more modern "reasonable prudence" standard, which appears to be the general direction of the law.[33] Regardless of which standard serves as the benchmark, measuring professional liability essentially involves weighing relevant and material evidence to determine whether a health care professional's knowledge and conduct met the applicable benchmark. Physicians whose conduct betrays an absence of knowledge about appropriate professional conduct risk liability for negligence; the risk of liability associated with the lack of knowledge is present even in states that also permit an affirmative defense linked to the inability to practice at the professional standard of care because of an absence of resources.[34] In other words, the inability to adhere to a standard may be a defense in a negligence claim; the lack of knowledge regarding the professional standard is not.

The Duty of Transparency: The Duty to Warn

A basic legal tenet embedded in the professional standard of care is the concept of physicians as "learned intermediaries," not only in relation to their patients, but also in relation to society as a whole.[35] The concept of a physician as a learned intermediary has arisen in the context of product liability cases involving prescription drugs and devices; in this context, the presence of a learned intermediary is not considered a basis for absolving a drug maker of product liability. Yet the concept of the learned intermediary underscores how society sees physicians, namely, as powerful sources and translators of information about risk in health and health care. As learned intermediaries, physicians become an essential force making understandable the wealth of information that increasingly guides health care practice.[36]

Thus, for example, from a legal perspective it is a physician, not a pharmacist or a manufacturer, who has a duty to warn patients regarding safety risks arising from adverse drug reaction incidents[37] or a medical device recall.[38] Indeed, so strong is the law's regard for physicians as learned intermediaries that, despite the duty of patient confidentiality, the law imposes a duty on physicians to warn third parties in certain cases about patient conditions that carry foreseeable risks to others. Courts have found—and in some jurisdictions, legislatures have created—a duty to warn third parties in cases involving the results of tests for sexually transmissible diseases,[39] genetics tests,[40] or threats of physical harm.[41] The law's regard for physicians as learned intermediaries and for their ability to communicate risk as a result of their superior knowledge, information and expertise is so strong[42] that legal scholars have concluded that even in an age of consumer-driven health care, courts will be averse to shifting the risk for information error from physician to patient.[43] Indeed the modern legal trend appears to be toward creating exceptions to physician/patient confidentiality principles in order to ensure physician disclosure of information necessary to public safety.[44]

The obligation of physicians to disclose information goes beyond information related to patient risk; it also emphasizes physicians' duty to disclose information regarding the risks that they themselves may pose as a result of physical or mental impairment to the manner in which they practice health care.[45] Thus, for example, a physician would have a duty to disclose the use of an unorthodox treatment that deviates from professional norms or evidence that his or her practice has deviated from expected norms. Courts have further held that physicians have a legal duty to disclose information related to financial conflicts and self dealing that could materially affect their patients' decisions on treatment.[46]

The Duty of Transparency: Informed Consent

The legal doctrine of informed consent is considered to be part of the foundation of modern health care practice.[47] Informed consent focuses on the communication of information by a medical professional to a patient. While standards vary from jurisdiction to jurisdiction, the doctrine focuses not only on the substance of the information given but also the manner in which the information is conveyed and the degree of understanding of the information that must be achieved.[48] Informed consent is more than transparency and disclosure; it is a degree of communication that ensures that a patient possesses the information necessary to make a meaningful decision about care, in accordance with the relevant standard used in any particular jurisdiction to measure the concept of "informed."[49]

The breadth of the information to be conveyed is a critical aspect of informed consent. It is not merely enough to inform a patient of the risks and benefits of one particular approach to care; the duty encompasses an obligation to apprise a patient of the risks and benefits of various alternatives in both diagnosis and treatment.[50] In other words, a physician must know not only the risks associated with his or her treatment choices, but the range of approaches to treatment and the risks associated with each possible course of care.

Protecting, Preserving, and Maintaining the Confidentiality of Information and Patient Medical Records

The confidentiality of patient information is a well known tenet of medical practice and health law, as is the proper management of information about patients. Medical records are understood to be a fundamental component of health care practice. As a result, the law imposes on health professionals a duty to manage information about patients properly, including creating and maintaining medical records in a manner that meets professional standards of conduct. Virtually all states have statutes governing the creation, maintenance, disclosure, and protection of medical records, and violation of these duties can result in both professional liability and the most severe sanctions by government agencies, including loss of license to practice.

In sum, how information is acquired, used, managed, preserved and disclosed is integral to the professional standard of care. As the breadth and depth of information has expanded, the importance of these health information duties correspondingly has grown. Health information duties extend far beyond an obligation to keep patient confidences and protect communications. Indeed, if anything, modern legal principles emphasize the role of physicians as learned intermediaries who, given their superior knowledge and access to information, incur disclosure obligations not only on behalf of their own patients but also of third parties (i.e., society at large), particularly in the case of information considered important to health and safety. As health information technology yields ever-greater information capabilities, these informational aspects of the professional standard of care can be expected to assume an increasingly important position in health care practice, with the result that the proportion of liability cases stemming at least in part from a failure of information—the failure to disclose information, act on information, or report information—may be expected to grow.

The Adoption of New Technologies

Technology constitutes a central "but often unappreciated" aspect of professional liability law; indeed, one scholar has noted that "the culture of technology drives medical liability" and further, that "the history of medical professional liability is a struggle between technological advances and injuries suffered when those advances fail."[51]

Technology creates two levels of possible liability exposure: the failure to adopt technology and the failure to use technology properly.

Failure of technology adoption

The first risk of liability arises when an industry lags behind reasonable expectations regarding the adoption and use of technology. The seminal case in this regard is *The T. J. Hooper*,[52] which, in focusing on the duty of tugboat owners to have operating radios on board their boats, says much about not only how courts weigh custom in determining if a profession has acted prudently, but also how the courts will weigh custom in an information context. The case concerned a tugboat accident in which the tugboats involved lacked operational onboard radios and thus proceeded onward despite broadcasted information about a violent storm. Despite evidence that operating onboard radios were coming into use but were not yet either a prevailing industry custom or required by law, Judge Learned Hand set the standard for framing questions of liability in relation to industry custom:

> Is it then a final answer that the business had not yet generally adopted receiving sets? There are, no doubt, cases where courts seem to make the general practice of the calling the standard of proper diligence. . . . Indeed in most cases reasonable prudence is in fact common prudence; but strictly it is never its measure; a whole calling may have unduly lagged in the adoption of new and available devices. [An industry] never may set its own tests, however persuasive be its usages. Courts must in the end say what is required; there are precautions so imperative that even their universal disregard will not excuse their omission.[53]

Equally important, the court's opinion noted two crucial pieces of evidence that would continue to guide courts in deciding questions of technology-related liability. The first was evidence of an emerging consensus within the industry regarding the value of adoption of the technology; indeed, the tugboats involved in the accident that led to the litigation had radios that failed to function. The second was evidence pointing to the relative low cost, and ease, of its adoption and maintenance.

Failure to adopt technology has served as the basis of much health law litigation, and key cases have focused on technologies whose aim is to improve the quality of information essential to proper patient care. In *Helling v. Carey*,[54] the Washington State Supreme Court held that the claim that glaucoma screening was not customary in patients under age forty was no defense in a malpractice action that involved the loss of vision to glaucoma by a woman in her thirties, and the corresponding failure by her physician to check her eye pressure using the practice's readily available screening technology. In *Washington v. Washington Hospital Center*[55] despite evidence that use of carbon dioxide monitors during surgery arguably was only just emerging as a standard of care, the court held that countervailing safety, cost, and utility evidence was sufficiently strong to serve as a basis for negligence liability.

There is little question that at this early stage in HIT, the value-based factors that propelled the case for adoption of technology in *The T. J. Hooper* and the *Helling v. Carey* case are missing. Furthermore, modern negligence practice turns far more on professional prudence than on a reasonable person standard. But as time passes, the cost of adoption of technology drops, and the prevalence of its adoption grows, there is a growing likelihood that physician performance will rise to the expectation that is enabled by properly used HIT.

Improper use of technology

Medical injury cases flowing from the improper use of technology are legion, even as advances in technology improve quality of care, they also can increase the risk of error and injury.[56] As technology becomes ever more cutting edge, so do legal expectations regarding its value in improving health care quality and patient safety.[57] At the same time, the added skills needed to use cutting edge technology may elevate the risk of liability in their own right. Indeed, errors associated with high-technology practice are thought to comprise a disproportionate percentage of preventable errors.[58]

In sum, HIT raises several legal issues in the broader context of health information. At what point will the level of knowledge and transparency enabled by HIT become a standard expectation of health professionals, thereby compelling adoption of the technology? Will diffusion have to reach a very broad level before HIT-enabled knowledge and transparency are the norm, or as in the *Washington Hospital Center* case, will public expectations trigger the obligation at a far lower level of diffusion? Clearly as long as the technology is costly and complex, the ability of the technology to act as the type of liability trigger seen in *The T. J. Hooper* and *Helling v. Carey* is lacking. But the pressure for and the growing speed of diffusion of HIT suggest that this time may not be as far off as some may believe.

Using HIT Adoption as a Tool for Rethinking the Legal Principles That Govern Health Care Practice

Given the role of information as a defining aspect of professionalism, as well as the degree to which HIT may improve the flow of information and promote greater skill, knowledge and transparency, it is perhaps inevitable that at some point the first liability cases attributable to the failure to have adapted to an information age will emerge. Indeed, while the news is full of spectacular breach of privacy stories, the most significant cases from a professionalism point of view may be those that have the effect of boosting the professional standard of care because of the level of knowledge that should have been enabled or conveyed but was not. This risk of liability is, of course, not limited to physicians. Ultimately it will reach hospitals and health care systems, which will face similar liabilities in their failure to adopt and make use of technology-enabled patient information. Indeed, one of the most seminal of all health law cases, *Darling v. Charleston Memorial Hospital*,[59] established the independent liability of hospitals as medical care institutions for the quality of their care. This concept means that as with physicians, hospitals face liability for failing to incorporate into their operations new technologies that are essential to patient safety and welfare. As technology advances the ability to use and share information, hospitals and other health care institutions can expect to share the same legal fate that awaits health professionals who resist change.

At some point, the broader question of liability reform arises as a means of spurring information use and transparency. In commenting on the slow pace of HIT adoption, Blumenthal and Glaser write of increasing "physician confidence in the law"[60] through the use of expert screening panels or specialized medical courts to eliminate frivolous cases alleging negligence in a medical informatics context.

It is indeed possible to envision a world in which advances in information technology spur far more ambitious rethinking of the legal principles that undergrid health care practice. As noted previously, the concept of medical liability is grounded in the individualized relationship between a physician and a patient. But health information technology enables a far greater depth and range of information and thus can be expected to create new expectations about health care quality information as well as the public transparency of that information. It is possible to imagine that, over time, this patient-centered or patient-specific concept of professional duty may give way to an alternative set of legal theories, ones grounded in broader concepts of generalizable duties toward society as a matter of consumer protection and patient safety. Under these more generalizable duty concepts, physicians may fairly be found to have duties, not only in relation to particular patients, but also in relation to the broader health care consumer public. The first glimmers of such a duty can be seen in the contractual requirements of payers such as Medicare or large health benefit service corporations that are beginning to condition provider participation or payment on the submission of quality data that in turn, is publicly disseminated to the covered group. Put more directly, it is not inconceivable that at some point a court, moved by health care in an age of information, will apply duty to warn and informed consent theory to both potential as well as actual patients. As a practical matter, that expanded duty to potential patients would, in turn, serve to accelerate and reinforce ongoing efforts to develop more and better information about the quality of health care and make that information widely transparent to the public.

Such a reformulation of medical care as a matter both of public welfare, as well as an individual patient duty, however, also may in turn intensify pressures for a replacement of the classic medical tort system with one of no-fault compensation. Under such an evolving view of the law, a technology-enabled health care system would adhere to strong public transparency and disclosure norms, while the direct and indirect economic costs of personal injury to any particular patient would be addressed through a no-fault compensation approach[61] as part of a broader social good. Legal obligations, embedded in broader consumer protection law and theory, thus would replace the older body of law that measures physician duty strictly in relation to individual patients. In such a reformed system, no-fault compensation would become the means of protecting the critical interests of individual patients, while broader concepts of consumer protection and safety would fundamentally reorient physicians' legal duties.

This basic shift in legal thinking would seem to be consistent with a world in which concerns about health care costs, quality and safety are high, in which patients receive half of the care known to be effective[62] and in which billions of dollars are spent on defensive efforts to shield from view the inner workings of health care. It is, perhaps, time to rethink the structure and alignment of legal theories as they apply to health care practice, as a means of moving the discussion forward. To the extent that HIT has such an effect, this result might turn out to be one of its greatest contributions.

Patient Data

Professionalism, Property, and Policy

The Issue

Imagine if public health authorities could rapidly check what percentage of all patients who had used a drug developed a particular medical problem. Such pharmaco-vigilance could identify dangerous drugs much more rapidly and effectively than is now possible. They could then warn physicians and the public, and develop guidelines on the drug's use, or recommend that the Food and Drug Administration (FDA) remove the drug from the market. Public authorities could use this information to evaluate the drug's safety in conjunction with clinical trials and other methods. Similarly, if researchers could compare how all or most patients with the same diagnoses nationally fared when treated with different therapies or regimes they would have a powerful tool to evaluate medical practice. They could identify superior, ineffective, and high-risk treatments. But, today, there is no national database with such information in it. As a result, many people die or are harmed before the risks of drugs or medical treatments are known.

The growth of electronic medical records and prescribing data is creating new opportunities to promote patient safety and protect the public. These records make quickly identifying medical risks and public health problems over a wide population possible. They could facilitate the evaluation of medical therapies and the performance of hospitals and providers. But an obstacle prevents this from occurring. Currently, organizations with access to patient data consider such records their property and often sell them for commercial uses. As a result, much of this data is not publicly available. Privatizing ownership of this data impedes its use for public purposes and restricts its beneficial commercial development as well.[1]

Today, an emerging industry taps patient data for uses beyond patient care, billing payers, or quality assurance, that is, for so-called secondary uses.[2] Organizations that have access to patient data from medical records, prescriptions, and billing records sell it to whoever they wish, on whatever terms they want, although they often follow voluntary industry guidelines on patient confidentiality and data stewardship. Academic medical centers, such as Boston's Massachusetts General Hospital and Brigham & Women's Hospital, are exploring how to commercialize the patient data they possess for sale to the government, biotechnology companies, insurers, consulting companies and investment analysts, publishers, and others.[3]

Typically, organizations with access to patient data do not sell it to end users. Rather, they sell it to firms that consolidate the data from several sources and market it for resale for particular uses. The consolidators obtain the data from organizations that care for patients (hospitals, physician group practices, and provider networks) as well as firms that sell medical products and services (e.g., pharmacies, medical device firms, and medical suppliers) and third-party payers. They also obtain data from the American Medical Association (AMA) and other physician organizations that identify physicians by license number, practice specialty, hospital affiliations, and location of practice. When put together this information allows the analysis of patient care over time, within and outside of hospitals, and across a range of providers.

The law has not resolved what property rights exist for patient data. The traditional rule made health care providers the owners of patient medical records but gave patients the right to access information in them, and restricted provider dissemination of the record or disclosure of information in it.[4] However, patients also had the right to ask health care providers to transfer their medical records to another doctor. The advent of electronic medical records makes dual record use or ownership much easier. It shifts the issues of ownership, control, and access from the medical records to the information in the medical record. Currently, patients have access to their medical records and to the information in them, as do providers and insurers. The law also protects patient privacy by restricting disclosure of certain patient information, but it does not give patients exclusive ownership rights to this information. Nor does the law grant exclusive property rights for patient data or control over it to the other parties that have access to this information.

Most people who have written about this issue have either favored maintaining the status quo and current default rules or they have advocated in favor of private ownership of such data (typically by the private firms that process it) with no restrictions on the firms' ability to sell it. The Heritage Foundation, for example, advocates private ownership of patient data and says that governmental authorities should have to purchase it on the same terms as all other parties.[5] The prevailing view is that the industry needs voluntary or private organization standards for confidentiality and stewardship of data (rather than government regulation) but that there should be no law on ownership of such data. A small group of scholars favors having patients own data about themselves.

In this chapter, I argue that the economic, legal, and moral reasons typically invoked to justify treating a resource as private property do not support doing so in this instance. Rather, they favor treating patient data as a public good that should be available to all. There is no need to create private property rights to encourage production of the data because it already exists. Organizations that provide patient care, sell medical services, and insure risk already collect such data to perform their work, either to comply with existing legal requirements, or to be paid. They will continue to collect the data whether or not they must disclose the information and whether or not they can sell it.

Medical professionalism also supports public ownership of patient data. A core value of medical professionalism is the promotion of patients' interests, public health, and the growth of medical knowledge rather than commercial interests. Many public health and safety benefits derivable from patient data require a database that is comprehensive and publicly available. Private ownership will fracture the database; make obtaining comprehensive data prohibitively expensive; and certainly restrict access. Furthermore, public access to patient data will not impede its beneficial commercial development. Private firms can use the data to develop products and services, display information in different formats, analyze the data, and sell these derived products. However, they will earn profits based only on the value that they add to the data, rather than monopoly profits, because others will also have access to the data.

Concern for patient privacy may appear to caution against public access. However, the risks to privacy are no greater when data is publicly owned and accessible than when private firms own the data. In both cases there need to be limits as to what information owners can reveal to ensure confidentiality. However, public oversight of such data is more likely to ensure patient confidentiality than when private entities own the data.

The Stakes for Medical Professionalism

The medical profession has an interest in ensuring that patient information is available to improve medical practice, even when this availability restricts opportunities for financial gain for physicians and medical institutions. Promoting the improvement of medical practice and patient welfare by making information on medicine publicly available is a value central to medical professionalism.

The AMA expressed this value in its 1847 Code of Ethics. It declared that it was unethical for physicians to "hold a patent for any surgical instrument or medicine."[6] The prohibition aimed to improve patient welfare by keeping vital information public rather than by privatizing it for individual gain. Contemporary law and medical ethics do not prohibit physicians from patenting inventions. Today we understand that patents can promote the growth of knowledge—rather than restrict it—by rewarding its creation. Current law grants patents to individuals for creative efforts that result in an original invention.

Nevertheless, making information public to improve patient welfare and medical practice remains a core value of medical professionalism. It underlies the profession's commitment to medical research, sharing knowledge through publications in professional journals, teaching and learning from colleagues, and engaging in peer review. The AMA articulated this value in its code of ethics in 2001 by stating, "A physician shall continue to study, apply and advance scientific knowledge, make relevant information available to patients, colleagues, and the public, obtain consultation, and use the talents of other health professionals when indicated."[7] Likewise, the Charter on Medical Professionalism (adopted by the American Board of Internal Medicine and the European Federation of Internal Medicine) requires physicians' commitment to create new scientific knowledge and to "participate in the development of better measures of quality of care."[8]

To fulfill these values the organized medical profession should promote the use of patient data to improve patient safety, medical practice, and public health by having such information owned publicly, rather than by private entities. Professional values favor public ownership of patient data because that will advance these goals better than private ownership. Only public ownership can guarantee that this information will be available to public authorities to promote public health and oversee medical care institutions and that it will be widely available for scholarly research and beneficial development. Public ownership is necessary to ensure the comprehensive database that is necessary for many important public uses.

Patient Data Markets

Organized medicine took the lead in developing a market for medical data. In the 1950s, the AMA commissioned Ben Gaffin and Associates to conduct the Fond du Lac marketing study (named after the Wisconsin community chosen to conduct the study because it reflected national demographics), to determine the influence of advertising, pharmaceutical detailing, peer opinion, and other factors on physician drug prescribing.[9] It distributed this study to the Pharmaceutical Manufacturers' Association and leading drug firms to encourage them to advertise in AMA journals and to form a partnership with the AMA on areas of mutual benefit. Then the AMA began to sell data to pharmaceutical firms that identified physicians by their license numbers, practice locations, and practice specialty. Pharmaceutical firms combined physician identifiers with prescription data from pharmacies that included the prescribing physician's license number.[10] They then tracked individual physician prescribing, patient drug use, and pharmaceutical sales for their own marketing and promotion purposes.[11]

Later, specialized firms—now referred to as medical information organizations (MIOs)—emerged to broker the purchasing and selling of medical data.[12] They purchased data from the AMA to identify physicians by their license numbers and other information. They purchased data from pharmacies and other firms that identified drugs dispensed by physician license number. MIOs combined the information they obtained from different sources to reveal prescribing patterns and market trends, and then sold it to pharmaceutical firms.[13] Pharmaceutical firms purchased the data from MIOs to track what drugs were prescribed by individual physicians and the sales by the medical detailers who visited them. They rewarded their medical detailers who were the best at promoting sales. They also used the data to target physicians for focused marketing efforts by detailers to change their prescribing practices and to evaluate the effect of their firm's advertising and marketing—as well as that of their competitors. The information collected also revealed the potential market for each class of drugs, the current sales of the pharmaceutical firm's own products and the products of competitors, and their respective market share.[14] Medical device manufacturers and other medical suppliers also purchased data for similar purposes.

More recently, MIOs have sold patient medical record data stripped of patient identifiers, referred to as anonymous or *"anonymized"* patient data. When combined with other data it reveals the diagnoses and profiles of patients for whom physicians prescribe various drugs and use various therapies. Pharmaceutical firms can thus promote drugs differently for each use and design different strategies to influence different physicians based on the way the physicians use drugs and the patients they serve. The marketing literature explains in detail the uses of such data.[15] Managed care organizations, hospitals, and regulatory authorities can use this information to identify inappropriate drug uses by physicians; to determine whether pharmaceutical firms market drugs for unapproved uses; and to assess the effect of different medical treatments on patient care. Other users of patient data include health service researchers, health economists, the FDA, and public health departments.

Firms also started to purchase patient data as a tool for their advocacy on policy issues. Regulatory agencies evaluate the safety and effectiveness of drugs and medical devices before approving their sale. Third-party payers, managed care organizations, and hospitals also evaluate drugs before placing them in their formularies. They evaluate medical devices before covering their costs or encouraging their use. They consider the devices' cost-effectiveness, their impact on patient health, and their value in relation to alternative products or treatments. Organizations that develop clinical practice guidelines also consider such information. Knowing this, firms that manufacture and sell medical products now purchase patient data from studies and use it to make their case for their products.

IMS Health, the largest supplier of medical information for market research, now markets patient data for policy advocacy.[16] It promotes data from its General Practice Research Database, for studies of cost, effectiveness, impact on health care spending, and medical outcomes. Its Web page says "Achieving a favorable endorsement from healthcare authorities is critical to ensure that new innovations reach the market and patients more quickly and are incorporated into appropriate guidelines of care."[17] It adds that product use is boosted by studies of "efficacy, safety, and cost-effectiveness as presented in peer-reviewed medical and scientific journals or via specialized conference[s]."[18] IMS also markets its consulting services, which produce "manuscripts and reviews for submission to peer-reviewed journals, clinical trial reports, expert reports, investigator brochures, abstracts, posters, slide sets."[19] In addition to policy advocacy, consulting firms, group purchase organizations, software vendors and other commercial enterprises purchase patient data for various commercial uses.[20]

The market for patient data is worldwide. IMS markets such data in over one hundred countries and in 2006, earned over two billion dollars in revenue.[21] It sells data to all major pharmaceutical and biotechnology companies.[22] In addition, medical information firms see the potential for a new industry of data warehouses, data exchanges, and data-related products and services.

Promoting Private Data Markets

Private foundations, government policy, and private firms all now promote private data markets in various ways. Numerous groups are developing voluntary standards for the sharing, aggregation, and use of private data. These efforts are encouraged by the Department of Health and Human Services' Office of the

National Coordinator for Health Information Technology. As part of this effort, in June 2007, the Agency for Healthcare Research and Quality (AHRQ) proposed the creation of a National Health Care Data Stewardship Entity to set uniform operating rules and standards for sharing and aggregating public and private sector data on quality and efficiency.[23] It assumed that private parties would hold the data and have no obligations to supply data to the national government or state authorities.

The responses of many groups commenting on the AHQR proposal explicitly opposed the idea of public ownership. The American Medical Informatics Association (AMIA) reiterated its position "that there be no central repository of aggregate data—whether at the national or regional level."[24] The Markle Foundation's *Connecting for Health* project stated that "A single data repository for aggregating and reporting quality data could fail to meet user needs, increase the risk of large scale privacy violations and undermine public trust."[25] Three private organizations, the National Committee for Quality Assurance, the National Quality Forum, and the Joint Commission, proposed that they operate the national stewardship entity and charge fees for their work. They said they would determine data control and ownership rights. In brief, they would decide what data would be public, and what access would be provided to datacontributors.[26] They explained that those "that have the most data. . . . must be assured that their data will be properly protected. . . . [and that those who contribute data] want to maintain a competitive advantage, based on the value of their data."[27]

Current and Potential Public Uses of Patient Data

Researchers have long used patient data from clinical trials to analyze the benefits and risks of drugs, medical procedures and therapies, as well as to analyze health care costs.[28] Data from patient records, however, makes possible similar evaluations at much less cost, yields continually updated information, and makes rapid learning possible. It provides information on populations and variables not included in clinical trials.[29] Analysis of patient data can help track adverse effects from drug use.[30] The FDA could use data on physician prescribing to contact physicians who are prime recommenders of drugs that have received a black box warning of their risks or to let them know when a firm withdraws a dangerous drug from the market. Such data can also help identify the extent to which physicians prescribe drugs for unapproved uses without scientific support.[31] Furthermore, patient data can help to identify public health and safety problems or to track differences in alternative organized health care systems.[32] Patient data can facilitate many administrative issues, including managing health care fraud.[33]

Patient data from electronic medical records are now mined for such uses.[34] The Veterans Health Administration has tapped its eight million patient records to evaluate medical treatments.[35] Kaiser Permanente has created a research database on its eight million enrollees. The Geisinger Health System of Pennsylvania uses its medical records of over two million patients to evaluate medical treatment and develop medical policies.[36] The Centers for Disease Control and Prevention (CDC) operates a program on vaccine safety using medical records on six million patients from seven health maintenance organizations (HMOs). The National Cancer Institute combines data from eleven health care systems for ten million patients. The Center for Medicare and Medicaid Services (CMS) plans to use data from its Medicare drug benefit program and other patient data to evaluate drug safety and effectiveness, and to track the prescription of drugs for unapproved uses.[37] Other federal programs also plan to use such information.[38]

Sometimes public authorities collect patient data and make it publicly available. The Centers for Disease Control's policy is to make its data freely available to the public for research. It says "The interest of the public . . . transcend[s] whatever claims scientists may believe they have to ownership of data acquired or generated using federal funds. Such data are in fact, owned by the federal government and thus belong to the citizens of the United States."[39] The state of California requires all hospitals to report patient discharge data to a state agency, which sells it to the public.[40] Yet, each of these databases is partial and small compared to the size a database of combined records across health care institutions and insurers nationally would be. Nor are these limitations overcome by the fact that MIOs sell data to academic researchers for scholarly studies.[41]

National, comprehensive, longitudinal patient data would permit analysis, research, the promotion of patient safety, and public health monitoring not possible today. However, Academy Health, the leading health-service research association, notes that health service researchers face obstacles in accessing data related to federal health programs and other population-wide health data. It therefore advocates the "development and dissemination of secondary health data as a public good."[42]

Why Ownership Matters

In 2006, the American Medical Informatics Association published a white paper of an expert panel that proposed a national framework for secondary use of patient data.[43] The AMIA asked the panel to address several questions, including "Who owns patient data and who has the right to access the data and for what purposes?"[44] The AMIA expert panel noted that there were problems with the way firms were currently using patient data.

> . . . some data usages . . . are neither well regulated nor subject to citizen oversight. Many recent regional efforts to establish health information exchanges face a business challenge to provide information utilities to the community at the lowest possible cost. . . . [S]tewards of these data exchanges and their business partners are exploring non-subscription models for revenue generation which frequently include selling clinically rich datasets to industries.[45]

Nevertheless, the AMIA panel recommended, "the focus needs to be on data access and control, not data ownership."[46] Yet, the property rights that the law accords in patient data will in large measure determine access and control over it. If legislation does not resolve the ownership of patient data, courts are likely to grant property interests to those who possess that data and preserve the status quo. Those who sell data will use contracts that do not allow purchasers to disseminate the data without their authorization and courts are likely to enforce these contracts.[47] The result will be limited access to fractured databases.

Moreover, while the AMIA advocates policies on data stewardship rather than property law, it does not include governmental health authorities as stakeholders with rights of access to patient data. However, it lists other stakeholders that should have access, including provider organizations, personal health record service providers, insurance companies, health data exchanges, and health data banks, as well as patients.[48] The AMIA says that data stakeholders should develop standards and guidelines for data stewardship. It assumes that data stakeholders—including firms that sell and purchase patient data—would develop a consensus on the oversight. The standards that these groups develop will reflect the interests of those who want to sell or purchase patient data, rather than the interests of patients or the public; moreover the standards do not legally bind individuals or organizations.[49]

Problems with Private Ownership:
The Example of Clinical Trial Data

Commercial firms use medical data as a resource to sell or as a tool to expand their markets and compete with rivals. As such, they often have an interest in restricting the data's availability to others and in mining the data only in so far as it promotes their economic gain. For example, Boston's Partners Healthcare (a joint venture of the Massachusetts General Hospital and Brigham & Women's Hospital) opposed the state of Massachusetts's plans to amass and sell data at the time Partners Healthcare was planning to commercialize its own data for such purposes.[50] The private ownership of data may thus undermine the public's interest in generating longitudinal data and national data, and in making such data accessible to public authorities as well as to private firms that can use it to promote beneficial therapies.

Clinical trial data provides an example. Firms that develop drugs and medical devices conduct clinical trials to demonstrate that their products are safe and effective in order to receive governmental approval for their sale. Conducting such trials is expensive and time consuming. Firms that undertake such costs would like to preclude competitors from using this data to develop generic versions of their products. Thus pharmaceutical and medical device firms sought international legal protection from competing firms using clinical trial test data that one firm had obtained for another firm's own drug or medical device approval process. They received protection in 1994 under the agreement on Trade-Related Aspects of Intellectual Property (TRIPS) of the World Trade Organization.[51] Delaying generic drugs from coming to market may be justified because the restriction rewards firms that invest in research. However, protecting the disclosure of clinical trial data also allows firms to suppress information about any health risks of their products. This has led some writers to criticize TRIPS and argue that test data should be public to ensure public safety.[52]

In the 1990s and the first years of the twenty-first century, there were numerous examples of pharmaceutical manufacturers that delayed the disclosure of their research data or suppressed it altogether when it revealed their product's health risks. Some pharmaceutical firms also published evaluations of drugs, which included only partial trial data, thus distorting what the trials demonstrated.[53] The International Committee of Medical Journal Editors believed such practices were inimical to good science and medicine and, in 2005, made the requirement that clinical trials be publicly registered before medical journals would review studies based on them for publication.[54] In 2007, Congress required that sponsors of clinically directive therapeutic trials (except phase I clinical trials) register the trial with the National Library of Medicine so that the information would be public.[55] However, regulatory agencies cannot use test data to evaluate competing generic products and manufacturers still have the ability to use test data exclusively for a period after marketing approval. There are also some other limitations on disclosure of test data. The tension between private commercial interests and public interests in disclosure of medical data persists in the conduct of clinical trials.

The use of patient data from clinical practice exhibits similar tensions.

Physicians, hospitals, insurers, and pharmaceutical and medical device firms have incentives to limit the availability of such data to insulate themselves from competition and oversight, or to gain an advantage over competitors. MIOs that purchase patient data have an interest in keeping it under their control. The first U.S. Copyright Act (enacted in 1790) did grant copyrights for compilations of information. Known as "sweat of the brow" protection, this was a different rationale for copyright than for creative work. But the 1976 Copyright Act required original selection of data in order for compilations to be protected.[56] And, in 1991, the Supreme Court held that copyright was not available for compilations unless they involved creativity.[57] Most patient data compiled in databases today is not a creative effort protected by copyright law in the United State or the European Union.[58] As a result, lawyers advise clients to select and arrange data in new formats to obtain copyright protection for such databases.[59] They draft contracts to limit the purchaser from disseminating data to others.[60] They also develop technology that restricts the use of information by those who do not have their permission.

The Economics of Public and Private Ownership
Public, Private, and Merit Goods

Economists distinguish between *public goods*, *private goods*, and *merit goods*. *Public goods* are goods that are both *non-excludable*—i.e., the benefits are available to all—and *non-rival*—i.e., individuals can use them without preventing others from also doing so. An example is information gathered for government purposes and maintained in public records. In contrast, with *private goods*, one person's use restricts use by others or diminishes the benefit that others receive. Examples include food and tangible resources.

Since the benefits of pure public goods cannot be restricted, individuals lack incentives to fund their production. Individuals can use public goods as free-riders, namely, without paying for their use. Furthermore, individuals that fund public goods cannot sell them for profit since others can use public goods without paying. On the other hand, public goods have significant value because their benefit can be widely shared and there is no need to ration their distribution. However, without collective financing, the production of public goods will be less than socially optimal.

Merit goods confer benefits on individuals, but also yield value for third parties. Education, for example, produces skills and knowledge for an individual who then benefits from new opportunities. At the same time, education also improves the welfare of third parties whom the trained individual serves. A free

market will produce fewer merit goods than is socially optimal. That is because
the cost of the merit good is borne by the individual receiving the good. He or
she has an incentive to pay only the economic value that the merit good creates
for him or her, not the economic value it has for society. For this reason, economists say the government should subsidize the production of merit goods.[61]

Some goods are not purely private or purely public. Non-tangible goods—
such as ideas, knowledge, and information—have aspects of public and private
goods. Legal rules often determine whether individuals can restrict others from
using these goods. For example, the law of intellectual property creates property interests for inventions and other intangible goods through granting patents
or copyrights. By protecting intellectual creation as property, the law creates
financial incentives to innovate.

What Kind of Good Is Patient Data?

Physicians and medical institutions now generate patient data for medical
records, prescriptions and billing. This is necessary to provide medical care, to
comply with regulations, and for them to receive payment. Thus, there is no
need to encourage organizations to record such data by making it a private good
and granting them the right to its exclusive use or sale.

Nevertheless, much of the data in patient records, prescriptions, and billing
statements is not currently publicly available. But such data could easily be
transformed into a public good if the government required organizations to
report it to public authorities.[62] The additional costs of such reporting will be
relatively small, particularly for electronically stored data. (Most insurers have
adopted electronic billing as the norm and the federal government promotes
the adoption of electronic medical information technology and the use of electronic medical records and electronic prescribing.)

Federal law already requires reporting and public disclosure of information in other contexts. For example, the Securities and Exchange Act of 1934
requires all firms that sell securities on stock exchanges to disclose all information that is relevant to investors deciding whether to purchase their stock.
Publicly traded firms must supply significant information on their operations,
finances, liability, market competition, market strategy, and their legal and
financial risk. In addition, the Medicare program requires hospitals to report
cost information on treatments and then analyzes it to revise reimbursement
payments. This information is also publicly available. The federal government
also makes census data publicly available and discloses data on economic trends.
Massachusetts, Maine, New Hampshire, and some other states already have all-
payer claims databases for health care.

The Choice of Private or Public Ownership:

Lessons from Commons and Anti-Commons

The law determines whether private parties or the public owns property and the scope of property rights.[63] Defining property interests has important social consequences. Private ownership sometimes encourages individuals to create, invest in, or care for the resources, thereby promoting the public welfare. At other times it does the opposite.

Public ownership sometimes produces the so-called *tragedy of the commons*.[64] If a non-renewable resource is publicly available and individuals pay no fee based on their individual use of it, individuals have no incentive to use the resource prudently and the resource is likely to be overused and depleted. This often occurs in commonly owned grazing fields and fishing grounds. Private ownership of the resource often precludes such a tragedy. Private owners bear the full benefit and cost of the resource and therefore have an incentive to limit its use to sustain its continued economic value and to invest in its protection and development. Similarly, management and regulation of the publicly owned resource can also preclude the tragedy.[65] Public management of the resource can sustain it by limiting its use and by making investments to develop the resource. Analysts frequently invoke the tragedy of the commons as grounds to favor private rather than public ownership.

However, private ownership can produce an opposite problem called "the tragedy of the anti-commons." When "multiple owners each have a right to exclude others . . . and no one has an effective privilege of use," they can stifle innovation and the effective use of any of the individual property.[66] When ownership of basic building blocks for innovations is divided among numerous parties, the cost of combining them may preclude their being used to create new inventions. Today individuals patent some biomedical processes and tools that are not valuable in themselves. Each such patent creates a monopoly for raw material needed to create a product thereby making the cost of end products much higher than if there was one owner.[67] As a result, private ownership may produce little or no benefit for the individual owners as well as for the public, because the value of it is realized only when it is combined with other patents and results in new down-stream uses later on.

Lori Andrews, a legal scholar who writes on genetic issues, has shown this anti-commons problem in the patenting of genetic sequences.[68] In recent years, companies have patented gene sequences associated with diseases that are important in genetic testing and research. Athena Neuroscience Inc. holds a patent on apolipoprotein E, a gene related to Alzheimer's disease.[69] Myriad Genetics was granted a European patent related to breast cancer that protects all methods for diagnosing the cancer that compare the patient's BRCA1 gene with the patented BRCA1 sequence.[70] Researchers searching for cures or treatments of genetic diseases will have to obtain rights from the patent owners of those gene sequences and the hundreds of genetic mutations of those genes that are also patented. Moreover, the U.S. Patent Trade Office requires that individuals who discover a gene should not develop products based on the gene or undertake mutual testing of the gene without the permission of those who hold patents on expressed sequence tags created from the gene. Negotiating such rights creates an obstacle to research on curing genetic diseases.

In a similar vein, private ownership of patient data would probably preclude its most valuable uses by fracturing population data.[71] If each patient had exclusive property rights to his or her medical data, the cost of collecting and using population data would be prohibitive.[72] Granting property rights in patient data to physicians, hospitals, or insurers would fracture the data into larger segments but still impose significant costs on collecting patient data and making use of aggregate data.

In principle, private firms could purchase data from multiple organizations and create population-wide databases. However, some organizations may benefit more from withholding data than from selling it. Hospitals and managed care organizations might prefer to avoid the negative publicity, regulatory oversight, loss of market share, or liability risk that revealing patient data might produce. Pharmaceutical and medical device firms do not have an interest in disclosing data that might reveal their products' risks for the same reasons.

Even if private MIOs developed comprehensive patient databases, they might sell comprehensive or nationwide data at prices that are unaffordable for public authorities. Such risks are significant because governmental and public health uses are likely to require comprehensive data, which will be more expensive than subsets of data that commercial firms purchase to promote their particular businesses. Furthermore, some organizations may earn more by selling data to one or a few purchasers exclusively than by making it generally available.

Private ownership of patient data can also lead to monopolistic practices. Patient data has value in part due to the information it provides, and in part due to its analysis, its presentation, and the services and products derived from the data. When patient data is privately owned, its owners can tie together the sale of data and the sale of related services and products. Such tie-ins restrict competition over the services, since no other firm has access to the data. This problem disappears if the data is publicly available and multiple firms compete in providing data analysis and related services and products.

Public ownership of data would stimulate the development of data-related services and products by making data readily available and precluding data monopolies. Entrepreneurs could add value to the data by organizing it in original ways, facilitating its use, or combining it in software or simulation models. Individuals and firms would have incentives to develop data-related services and products because they could sell these.

Privacy as a Restraint on Use of Patient Data

Physicians obtain information about patients in order to diagnose and treat their medical problems. This information could be used to the detriment of patients. A canon of medical ethics is that physicians should act in their patients' interests. A related principle holds that physicians should not disclose confidential patient information.[73]

State laws generally prohibit health care providers and institutions from disclosing confidential patient information to third parties, except insurers, without the consent of patients. However, sometimes a statute or court order requires disclosure.[74] Sometimes individuals can use patient information for secondary uses in ways that do not compromise confidentiality.[75] For example, it is possible to evaluate medical care by examining patient data for a large group of patients without knowing their individual identities.

There are limits on patient confidentiality and patients' control over their medical information. Society has an interest in public health that sometimes conflicts with patient confidentiality. For instance, the law requires that physicians and health care institutions report certain communicable diseases. Physicians are also sometimes required to breach confidentiality to protect identifiable individuals from clear and direct harm.[76] Furthermore, third-party payers have a right to certain patient information to ensure the appropriateness of physician and patient claims for reimbursement. Today, physicians and researchers make use of information from patient records to evaluate medical treatment. Health care institutions and managed care organizations use patient information to oversee the quality of medical care.

Since 1996, the federal Health Insurance Portability and Accountability Act (HIPAA) has regulated the disclosure of patient information by designated entities. However, HIPAA allows a significant amount of disclosure and sale of patient data. The HIPAA amendments in 2003 allow covered entities to share patient medical information with health-care-related businesses (including employers, drug and insurance companies, marketing firms, accountants, banks and financial service companies, data warehousers, medical transcribers, data processing firms, consumer reporting agencies, pharmacies, and legal services).[77]

It also allows the sharing of information that does not identify the individual patient's identity.[78]

As a result today many medical organizations share confidential patient data with health-care related businesses or sell such data. They freely sell patient data that does not state the patient's identity to a wide range of entities. As was mentioned above, such data is often referred to as *"anonymized"* data, or sometimes as *"deidentified"* data. Yet even with such data, there are risks to patient privacy. A patient medical record that does not state the patient's identity may still indicate their physician, pharmacy, hospital, zip code, or insurer. By combining this information with other information that is either public or purchased from private parties, it may be possible to identify the patient.

The legal protections that historically have protected individuals from physicians, insurers, banks, and others disclosing their personal information have not arisen from the law recognizing such information as the individual's property. Rather privacy laws and other principles have supplied the governing standards.[79] Nevertheless, some privacy advocates argue that the best way to ensure patient confidentiality is to designate patient data as the property of patients and to prevent others from using the data without patients selling them rights to the data.[80] Such an arrangement would require creating a costly complex infrastructure to oversee data markets.[81] Moreover, granting individuals property rights to their personal data is not a particularly good way to protect privacy. Individuals may be willing to sell data to one purchaser for a particular purpose, but restrictions to selling for other purposes will be very hard to enforce after the sale, particularly if the purchaser sells or otherwise transfers the data to others. Monitoring compliance with initial restrictions to future purchasers will be difficult.[82]

In any event, there may be risks of unauthorized disclosure of personal information both when private firms and the public own such data. Under both forms of ownership there need to be measures to safeguard privacy. Firms already obtain and sell patient information. So making this information, or some of it, publicly available would not create significant privacy problems that do not already exist.

In fact, public reporting and ownership may offer greater privacy protections than currently exist. The law could limit firms from selling data. These legal authorities could then ensure that no data is publicly released that does not comply with privacy safeguards. Public authorities are more likely to implement such policies than private firms because they do not have a profit motive to sell confidential information, while private firms do. In addition, when the data is publicly owned, it will be overseen using a uniform standard, which is not the case when it is sold by private organizations, each of which may have their own policies and operating methods.

Furthermore, public ownership of patient data is likely to allow greater oversight on its use to protect privacy than federal regulation of the use of privately owned patient data. The U.S. Constitution's Fifth Amendment restricts the government from *taking* private property without compensating the owner. Courts have held that regulation of property often constitutes a *taking* of the property because it restricts rights to the property's use.[83] As a result, sometimes the government cannot regulate property use because it lacks the financial means to compensate the property owner.

What Data to Make Public and How to Do It

The details of what kind of data to make public, how to implement data reporting, and what measures should be put in place to ensure patient confidentiality require further work. However, these issues are already being discussed by the health information industry and providers as they collect and sell patient data today and as they explore sharing data in the future among private markets. Their analysis and conversations can be a starting point for examining these issues. Public reporting will initially be restricted by what data is available in electronic format. Currently, billing records generally are in electronic format, but many providers do not yet use electronic medical records or electronic prescribing. As standards for electronic medical records evolve this too will affect what and how data should be reported and by whom.

Here I offer some preliminary suggestions as to what parties the law might require to report information and what data they should report. California provides a model. It requires all hospitals in the state to report data on patients within thirty days of discharge. Hospitals report patient diagnosis, therapy, drug use, and other information about patient care and medical conditions without identifying the patient. California makes this information available for all hospitals in a single database for a small fee.

Federal law could require all United States hospitals to report the same data as California does to the Department of Health and Human Services (DHHS) or to a public authority created for this purpose. It could expand hospital reporting to include ambulatory care data as well as inpatient data. Hospitals should report patient discharge data in a way that allows analysis of patient care by hospital, physician, diagnosis, procedure, therapy and drugs prescribed. Other medical institutions (ambulatory care surgery centers, rehabilitation facilities, nursing homes, and community health centers) should be required to report similar data.

Pharmacies and all other individuals and entities that dispense drugs (including pharmaceutical benefit managers, clinics, and physicians and nurses that dispense drugs) should report the drugs they dispensed by dosage, provider ID number, and diagnosis when this information is available. Dispensers that submit data to third-party payers for reimbursement should provide the same data to the DHHS at the same time. Firms not reimbursed by third-party payers should also report dispensing data monthly.

Providers should submit the same patient information to the DHHS as they do to third-party payers when seeking payment. In addition, providers should submit current patient profile data to the DHHS on a quarterly basis. All data should protect patient confidentiality by not revealing the patient's identity. However, providers should submit their data with their own tracking number so that it is possible to analyze the care that patients received from them over time by analyzing quarterly reports. Third-party payers, managed care organizations, and Employee Retirement Income Security Act (ERISA) self-funded health benefit plans' administrators should report patient data, dispensing data, and billing information that they receive from their providers and from dispensing organizations.

To ensure confidentiality procedures should be worked out for reporting information that eliminates patient identifiers before the data are reported to the DHHS. In addition, the DHHS should review submitted data and scrub it to eliminate patient identifiers before releasing it. The DHHS should make patient data available to the public, perhaps charging modest user fees.

Limitations

Patient data currently available has significant limitations for the purpose of promoting public health and patient safety.[84] For example, hospital data is typically based on billing information rather than on medical records, and on individual episodes of care, rather than by individual patients. Often data available from patient records is not linked to billing information. It is thus difficult to track information on patients across health care settings and over time. Furthermore, there is no uniform system of collecting or recording such information, there are multiple formats, and differing software complicates working with data across institutions. Creating, maintaining, and administering such databases is difficult and costly. These are significant impediments to effective use of patient data for patient safety and health promotion. However, these affect implementation, not the value of such data or the arguments in favor of public reporting and ownership.

Some implementation problems may be resolved as technology develops that integrates patient records, prescribing information, and billing, and as technology for managing data develops. However, requirements for public reporting are likely to facilitate resolving these problems. The use of electronic data has developed rapidly and effectively where governmental policies or large private institutions have set a single standard of information that must be collected and the technology that must be used. Several European countries have developed electronic record keeping and are ahead of the United States. France, for example, has a uniform system for recording patient data. In Asia, Taiwan also has developed a uniform electronic system for patient records.[85]

In the United States, the Veterans Health Administration is a national leader in electronic record keeping in large part because it has been able to require a uniform universal standard across all facilities and providers. Other leaders in collecting and using patient information are large, integrated HMOs and health care systems, such as Kaiser Permanente and the Geisinger Health System. But for much of the United States, competing insurers, and private health care institutions create incompatible standards and policies on collecting data. Furthermore, the absence of legal reporting requirements and standards for electronic record keeping and technology also adds complexity. Some of these problems would disappear or become much easier to address if the federal government set standards for what must be collected and reported, and also the technological standards that must be used for electronic medical databases.

Sheila M. Rothman, Natassia M. Rozario, and David J. Rothman

Chapter 6

The Impact of Information Technology on Organ Donation

Private Values in a Public World

The most intractable problem facing kidney transplantation over the past several decades has been an unrelenting shortage of organs. Transplant patients not only live longer than patients on dialysis but also enjoy far better lives. Surgical techniques and anti-rejection drugs have improved to the point that 95 percent of kidney grafts from living donors and almost 90 percent from cadaveric donors survive the one-year mark.[1] A forty-year-old patient has close to a 90 percent chance of surviving five years post transplant.[2] The indispensable but missing element remains the organ. Some 80,130 people are now on the waiting list for a kidney transplant.[3] Every year, over 4,000 people have died waiting for a kidney.[4]

Not surprisingly, patients with end stage renal disease (ESRD) pursue a variety of strategies to obtain an organ. They may ask either close or distant relatives to serve as living donors; they may ask friends, co-workers, and fellow parishioners about the possibility as well. And, to the point of this inquiry, they may also turn to the Internet. The tactic is certainly novel and its practice and implications are barely understood. Without question, there are some very negative aspects to the venture, raising considerations that are at odds with ethical, legal, and medical standards. But at the same time, the use of the Internet has broadened the scope of possibilities for a patient in search of a transplant and may well reflect a new and vital aspect of social relationships. The purpose of this chapter is to explore both perspectives so as to understand better the emerging relationship between information technology and medical professionalism.

Scarcity in Medicine: The Dialysis Story

From one perspective, the impact of the use of new information technology for organ donation has been markedly retrogressive. Patients going online to request a body part invoke a set of values that once were central to medical decisions about the allocation of scarce resources but have subsequently been rejected. The best case in point comes from an earlier history of another technology used to treat ESRD, that is, kidney dialysis. Through the 1960s and 1970s, dialysis machines were life-saving but in very short supply. The effort then to capture a time slot on a machine bears an intriguing resemblance to the effort today to obtain a kidney.

The dialysis story is well known and begins with Belding Scribner at the University of Washington in Seattle. In 1960, he devised a special shunt that allowed patients to be attached on a long-term basis to a machine that served as a surrogate kidney and cleansed the body of waste. Patients who went on the dialysis machines lived; those without access died. The difficulty was that there were far too few machines to treat even the Seattle patients with ESRD, forcing the University of Washington team to make life or death decisions case by case. The physicians were unwilling to bear that burden, on the grounds that each doctor would be, and had to be, an advocate for his own patients. Accordingly and at their own initiative, the physicians established a lay committee of ordinary citizens to make the allocation decisions.[5]

The lay committee went about its work by first interviewing all the dialysis candidates who had been certified by the medical team as in need of the dialysis technology. The committee members then developed the criteria for making their decisions. They gave preference to the married over the unmarried, to couples with children over couples who were childless, to the employed over the unemployed, the law-abiding over the criminal, the community participant over the loner, the younger over the older, and the churchgoing over the non-churchgoing. As one contemporary law review article summed up the standards, "The Pacific Northwest is no place for a Henry David Thoreau with bad kidneys."[6]

Although reaction was slow in coming, the Seattle proceedings sparked very negative responses. The idea of a "Who Shall Live" committee was fundamentally at odds with American values. It took time, but a small group of dialysis patients organized themselves to press for federal funding for dialysis, and they met with extraordinary success. Medicare provided special coverage to ESRD patients, in effect giving national health insurance to everyone with diseased kidneys. Once federal payments were in place, the number of dialysis machines and dialysis centers, including for-profit centers, proliferated and shortages disappeared. In all, the dialysis experience made clear, first, that rationing life-saving resources was unacceptable. (By contrast, the British National Health Service had no problem setting and maintaining age limits for access to dialysis.) Second, the use of social criteria to distribute scarce medical resources was, at its core, unfair and inappropriate.[7]

How curious, then, that a dependence on social criteria rejected in kidney dialysis should be revived in kidney donation. For, as we shall see, this is precisely the impact that follows from the use of information technology (IT) to obtain an organ. IT restores to prominence the very standards that were rejected for allocating use of dialysis machines.

Kidney Donation and the Family Network

It is well recognized that the shortage of cadaveric kidneys for transplant has persisted despite a variety of regulatory and educational efforts. The enactment of Federal Required Request regulations, whereby hospitals must ask family members of a deceased patient whether they would allow organ donation has had little effect; so too, advertising slogans and publicity campaigns have not drastically increased kidney donation rates. At the same time, the superiority of transplant over dialysis as measured by patient morbidity, mortality, and quality of life has become even more evident. Ideally, if a kidney were available, an ESRD patient would undergo transplant without ever going on dialysis.

Not surprisingly, then, once a patient is diagnosed with ESRD the transplant team will immediately ask whether a spouse, child, relative, or friend might make an organ donation. The team will explain that from the perspective of the donor, the long-term risks of living with one kidney are minimal; some discomfort and a period of recuperation will follow kidney removal, but now that laparoscopic rather than open field surgery has become standard, recovery is quick and the resulting scar, barely visible. From the perspective of the recipient, there will be no waiting period for an organ (which otherwise averages two to three years), and the organ retrieved will be in optimal condition. Not surprisingly, then, about 40 percent of all kidney transplants now use organs from living donors.[8] Because cadaveric donation rates have remained relatively static for several decades, the percentage of living donors for transplantation is certain to increase in the future.

Donors come primarily from the immediate family. In 2006, 67 percent of the 6,432 living donations were parent to child, child to parent, sibling to sibling, or spouse to spouse; "other relatives" made up 7.4 percent of the donations. Friends, neighbors, and other persons not related to the kidney recipient represent 22.4 percent (see table 6.1).[9] Although there is no data on the precise

Table 6.1   **Living Organ Donation, 2006, by Donor Relationship**

Relations	Number	Percentage
Parent	658	10.23%
Child	1,145	17.80%
Sibling (includes identical twin, full sibling, and half-sibling)	1,715	26.66%
Other relative	478	7.43%
Spouse	788	12.25%
Anonymous	68	1.06%
Paired exchanges/nonbiological (living and deceased) donor exchange	96	1.49%
Other unrelated directed	1,438	22.36%
Not reported	46	0.72%
All donors	6,432	100.00%

Source: Organ Procurement Transplant Network, "Living Donor Transplants by Donor Relation" (April 25, 2008), http://www.optn.org/latestData/rptData.asp (accessed from the OPTN/UNOS Web site on April 30, 2008).

relationship between these persons and the recipients, patients probably turned first to neighbors, friends, and fellow employees. Strangers are likely to be a last resort, but appeals to them are increasing—which brings us to the Internet.

Enter the Internet

Numerous Web sites are now serving as a channel for organ donation requests. Some serve a particular individual: helpmygrandpa.com, or, donationforcynthia .com. Others follow ethnic or religious lines: halachicdonors.com. Still others are more universal in orientation, and one that has attracted particular attention is matchingdonors.com.

The Web site was designed in 2003 by Paul Dooley, a businessman who had earlier designed an Internet program to help employers recruit employees. Dooley charged the employers an annual fee of $295 to list their available positions on his Web site, and through advertising brought the site to the attention of young people, especially college graduates, seeking jobs. The venture worked—the site was successful and profitable. Shortly thereafter, Dooley's father was diagnosed with ESRD, and Dooley immediately put his Internet knowledge to work to get him a kidney. His father's physician joined him on the project, and together they fashioned a site that replicated for organs what Dooley had done for employment.[10] Would-be recipients of kidneys pay the fees: lifetime membership costs $595; a three-month membership, $441; a thirty-day

Table 6.2   **Categories of Social Worth Used by Patient Profiles on matchingdonors.com**

Category	Percentage of patients who used social worth category*
Family values	69%
Economic factors	35%
Religious beliefs	38%

n = 100 postings, collected between February 2005 and March 2006

*Totals exceed 100 percent because postings often invoked more than one value.

membership, $295; and a seven-day trial membership, $49. There is no charge to would-be donors. At the end of 2009, the site listed 7,416 prospective donors and 249 patients.[11]

To understand how potential recipients attempt to persuade strangers of their worthiness to receive an organ, we analyzed the first hundred personal profiles on matchingdonors.com between February 2005 and March 2006. The profiles emphasized the very same social criteria that were once regarded as inappropriate in dialysis allocation decisions. Family values, economic factors, and religious beliefs were all invoked to demonstrate merit for a transplant (see table 6.2).

The texts composed by would-be organ recipients, like their counterparts in online dating and open-adoption appeals, function as a form of promotional discourse or "commodification of self" that involves the "promoting or 'selling' of selves" and "attracting or 'buying' of others."[12] In all these arenas, idealized self-identities are offered in terms of measures of desirability (age, physical attributes, personalities, interests). In dating, men and women emphasize personality, appearance, income, and receptivity to adventure; in open adoption, prospective parents highlight family values, strong traditions, financial stability, and societal contributions. In the online transplant world, the model version of self has some of the qualities of the dating entries but even more of the open adoption ones.[13] In all three domains, the presentations serve as a "sorting mechanism."[14] Potential takers can evaluate the purported characteristics of the persons who have posted their narratives and then select among them.

Most would-be organ recipients tried to establish their social worth by emphasizing family values. Almost seventy of the one hundred postings mention the patient's family role as parent, grandparent, or significant other. (Occasionally, an Internet appeal mentioned that no one in the individual's family circle was available to donate, but the issue was usually passed over without explanation.) When a would-be recipient was older, the plea typically took the form of gaining more time with grandchildren and being able to watch them grow up.

> "My father is the backbone of our family and his illness has managed
> to create heartache within each of us."
> "I hope and pray that there is someone out there who wants to help me
> see my grandchildren grow up."
> "I am now in need of a kidney to enable me to continue my life with
> my husband, children, and grandchildren."
> "I have one daughter who is now expecting a baby and I want to live
> to see my grandchild grow up."

Profiles also invoked economic worthiness, coupling it with social contributions. One-third of the postings mention occupation, with kidney patients often noting the fulfillment their job brings to them and to the people they serve—all of which would be lost unless an organ donation was forthcoming.

> "The [battered] women and [abused] children that come to me for help
> mean a lot to me and as much as I want to be there for them, it gets
> harder and harder because I feel weaker and weaker every day."
> "I am hopeful of receiving a transplant so that I can return to [my oph-
> thalmology] profession that I have trained to be a part of and where
> I have received my greatest pleasures in life—saving the eyesight of
> the poor and disadvantaged."

In effect, the patient is promising to repay society for the investment made. It is also worth noting that transplant teams themselves take great pride in announcing that many of the kidney recipients returned to work, using employment as an index of success ("he was well enough to rejoin the labor force") and also as a justification for transplant ("yes, it is expensive but the recipient is now contributing to the common weal and paying taxes").

Finally, more than a third of postings highlighted religious values, trying to appeal across denominational lines.

> "I love God so much. The Lord is my priority."
> "Donation will allow me to accomplish what God intends for me with
> my family and those who surround me."
> "I need a kidney to continue to do God's work . . . I believe He sends
> people to meet the needs of His children."
> "You will be blessed by God."

The invocation of social criteria by these patient profiles stands in marked contrast to the rejection of social criteria in the Seattle dialysis experience. There, the ultimate resolution was to make the allocation decision regardless of whether the patient was a parent or grandparent, well employed, or a devoted parishioner. Online, however, these are the criteria emphasized in the hope that they will persuade potential donors not only to give an organ but also to help them decide to whom to give. Status and position, not length of time on a waiting list or gravity of illness, become the decisive factors in determining whose online profile makes the patient most deserving of an organ.

Organ Donation and New Social Networks

These negative aspects noted, the shift to Internet organ solicitation also reflects a new and expanded definition of community. As a number of analysts propose, the Internet represents a new mechanism for accumulating and dispensing social capital. Seeking a donor online is part of the same trend that brings singles to Internet dating sites and want-to-be parents to open-adoption sites. For all of these individuals, choices are expanded and worthy ends achieved by using Internet sites. Matches are made from an enlarged pool, increasing the likelihood of satisfactory outcomes.

Social capital, as defined by Robert Putnam, "refers to the collective value of all 'social networks' and the inclinations that arise from these networks to do things for each other."[15] Traditionally, network formation, solicitation, and implementation centered on the village and neighborhood. Over time, however, geographically focused networks have given way to more dispersed ones. The relationships now underlying social capital reflect what has been called, "networked individualism." In this new system, people connect through choice, not by space.[16]

The shift has been driven conspicuously, but not exclusively, by the Internet. It has made it convenient, indeed simple, for people to connect regardless of place of residence or intimate knowledge of each other. It has allowed people to maintain and strengthen old ties while at the same time creating opportunity to forge new ones. As Manuel Castells notes: "The emerging pattern is one of self-directed networking, both in terms of social relationships and in terms of social projects. It does not substitute for face-to-face sociability or for social participation. It adds to it. . . . Thus, the Internet is an appropriate tool for networking, and for self-directed horizontal communication."[17]

The Pew Internet and American Life Project 2006 Report on "The Strength of Internet Ties" substantiates these claims. The Report presents findings from two daily tracking surveys on Internet use among Americans: the Pew Social

Ties Survey and the Pew Internet Project Major Moments Survey. Both used a sample of 2,200 adults, aged eighteen and over. The surveys examined the impact of the Internet on relationships among friends, relatives, and co-workers, paying particular attention to how online resources affected options around major life decisions, including serious illness and chronic medical conditions. Both surveys found that respondents used the Internet to activate their social networks when they needed help, and that the Internet built rather than eroded social capital. Internet users could draw on a larger social network than non-users.[18] As the report concludes: "Americans are in an era where they may have only one or two extremely close relationships, but dozens of core and significant ties. This means rather than relying on a single community, people do better when the actively seek out a variety of appropriate people and Web resources for different situations."[19] In this frame, the Internet connects people in need of support to a multiplicity of resources and experts.

These trends have obvious relevance to living donation. Patients seeking an organ can look beyond their close relationships for other connections. The Internet makes it possible for them to go outside of local institutions in their communities and seek potential donors who would otherwise be beyond reach. Forty years ago, would-be recipients of organs turned almost exclusively to their family, usually the immediate one but sometimes the extended one. Now, they will turn not only to high school or college friends scattered around the country but also to members of common interest network clubs, or even total strangers. Face-to-face solicitation has given way to Internet connectivity.

Internet solicitation for organs may have yet another characteristic, beyond the values promoted and the social capital gained. The Internet appears to decrease the levels of personal discomfort experienced by would-be organ recipients as they make their requests for help. In effect, they cast their nets more widely through the Internet not only because of its connectivity but also its impersonality. The idea of reciprocity has different meanings online and offline, which becomes manifest when comparing "the asking process" in the two contexts. Online postings for an organ typically adopt a bold and deliberate display of need and make an unqualified and explicit request for an organ. On the other hand, patients seeking an organ from an intimate circle of friends and family are frequently reluctant to make the request and to make known the gravity of their medical condition, tempering both in a variety of ways. It is not unusual for the would-be donor to be far more eager to give an organ than the would-be recipient is to receive. Certainly, some ESRD patients are unsparing in their demands of their intimates. But reticence appears even more common. It seems easier to ask a stranger to undergo the pains of donation than a family member. There is less guilt involved, and possibly, less fear of the ensuing obligations.

In our field work with organ donors and recipients, patients' reluctance to ask for an organ was often striking. Between July 2005 and May 2006, we interviewed and then accompanied fifteen potential recipients and twenty potential donors to their initial evaluation appointments with members of a transplant team, including a nephrologist, a surgeon, a social worker, a financial coordinator, and a transplant coordinator. (The study received Institutional Review Board (IRB) approval, and all participants provided informed consent.) Among the potential recipients in our study, five out of fifteen expressed either guilt or hesitation about either asking a loved one for an organ or accepting one when the offer was unsolicited. As our field notes describe it (with some details altered so as to protect the anonymity of the patients):

> Patient is a forty-five-year-old man, suffering from ESRD and is currently on chemodialysis. He was diagnosed two years ago. The patient has ten siblings and twenty-seven potential donors.
>
> Patient was extremely reluctant to accept an organ from any one of them. During his interview with the social worker, he joked that his family "did not leave him alone and would not stop bothering him." Four of his sisters called him that morning before his appointment to make sure that he was okay. He was not used to the attention. He missed the independence he had prior to his diagnosis and felt enormously guilty for how reliant he already had become upon his family. He did not want to ask them for any more favors, let alone an organ.
>
> [Field Note, August 2005]

> Patient is a fifty-five-year-old man. He is considering the possibility of a living organ donation from his younger brother, who is forty-four. During his evaluation, the patient expressed reluctance to accept his brother's kidney. His brother's wife was nervous about his brother going through with the donation. The patient was also anxious about the risks associated with the nephrectomy given the family history of diabetes. During his evaluation with the nephrologist, he said, "He's my little brother. . . . That's the last thing I want is for my brother to give up his kidney and then to get diabetes."   [Field Note, September 2005]

> Patient is a fifty-five-year-old woman suffering from kidney disease and was recently diagnosed with Hep(atitis) C. She was not on dialysis but was interested in learning more about the option of transplantation. She had overcome remarkable obstacles, including a twenty-seven-year

addiction to crack and cocaine and a ten-year period of being homeless. It was only at the age of forty-one that things began to change in her life. She returned to school, got married, and started her own non-profit working with children of drug-addicted parents. At the moment when everything finally seemed to coalesce, her health started to deteriorate. During her evaluation, several members of the transplant team inquired about her husband as a potential donor. They had met him before and were aware that he was the one who took care of her when she got sick. To the team, it seemed that he was the most obvious candidate to donate an organ. To the patient, however, the idea of having her husband donate was unsettling. When the social worker asked about the possibility of her husband donating, she said that she was unsure at that point. When the nephrologist asked about potential donors, she was reticent about providing her husband's name and seemed more interested in waiting it out for a cadaveric transplant.   [Field Note, December 2005]

Patient is a forty-nine-year-old woman with ESRD. She was interested in getting listed for a cadaveric organ. Both her husband and her sister wanted to donate. However, the patient seemed uncomfortable about using a living donor. While her sister "really wanted to donate," the patient was worried about the toll that surgery and recovery would take on her sister's family. When the nephrologist asked about the possibility of using her sister as a donor, the patient's immediate response was, "But she has two little ones." Her husband accompanied the patient during the evaluation. At one point, sensing that the wife was somewhat hesitant about proceeding with a living organ transplant, the husband said, "If you are going to go through with this, it is better to give it your best shot the first time."   [Field Note, February 2006]

Patient is a forty-eight-year-old man, who has persisted on dialysis for ten years and has refused all offers made by family and friends to donate. During his evaluation for a transplant, when asked about potential living donors, he responded, "No . . . I would never ask anyone that . . ." One of his friends had repeatedly offered to donate almost to the point of making him feel guilty for declining the gesture. The patient, nonetheless, emphasized that he would not feel comfortable having a loved one undergo the surgery.   [Field Note, March 2006]

Observing the process of living organ donation thirty years ago, the sociologist Roberta Simmons described in vivid detail the anxiety associated with asking a close family member for a transplant. She found that sixty percent of the recipients reported some guilt "at asking a relative to donate" and 28 percent reported a lot of the guilt." Simmons also noted the "considerable constraint" among patients to communicate their need for a donor among loved ones: "The norm expressed by a high percentage of the patients is that one should not ask for a kidney, one should wait for a volunteer."[20] Requests were often more veiled than explicit; kinship ties in many families can be highly fragile and unable to withstand open insult. Thus, the indirect request by the patient allows potential donors to evade replying and protects both parties from the consequences of rejection, including mutual embarrassment.[21]

These considerations disappear in an arena where direct obligation and existing emotional ties are absent. It is less challenging to openly ask something of a stranger than of an intimate. As the sociologist Felicia Wu Song observes, trust in a virtual community approximates the kind of reciprocity that George Simmel depicted in "The Stranger."[22] "The appeal of the stranger . . . is a function of the stranger's possession of (1) an apparent objectivity, and (2) a potential for mobility."[23] Accordingly patients may be more willing to solicit online precisely because the stranger "lacks personal ties that can prejudice perception."[24] The stranger has an "open mind" and is unaware of the personal details of the patient's life that could dissuade the person from donation. More, in terms of "potential for mobility," patients may be comfortable with online solicitations because the online community members can "disappear at any moment." In this context, even the most personal acts occur within a "structure of loose ties" and "quick compassion." In other words, after the stranger donates his kidney, the recipient, accurately or not, may believe that the donor "comes today and is gone tomorrow." The recipient is also not burdened by the worries and guilt that come with accepting a kidney from a loved one.[25]

The Downside of Online Organ Procurement

Recognizing these more positive considerations of online solicitation, we still conclude that the practice of going online to seek a donor carries many dangers. First, by the very nature of Internet communication, the potential for deception increases. Research on Internet dating fully documents the phenomenon. In one study, 90 percent of participants admitted to lying on the Internet; another report found that individuals actually regretted being honest online because the posting was not as effective as it might have been.[26] The anonymity of the Web sites and the Internet also provides users with unmatched opportunities for creativity with self-portrayal. As social scientist, Sherry Turkle, observes: "In cyberspace, it is well known, one's body can be represented by one's own textual description . . . The fact that self-presentation is written in text means that there is time to reflect and edit one's composition. . . . The relative anonymity of the life on the screen . . . gives people the chance to express often unexplored aspects of the self."[27] It is likely, then, that neither potential donors nor potential recipients of organs will be forthright and accurate in their personal information and intentions, which may well produce unexpected and devious situations involving illegal acts as well as physical and psychological harms.

Second, Internet recruitment carries too many opportunities for illegal practices, including the sale of an organ. It is one thing if covert exchanges of funds occur between siblings, but we may not want to institute a system that allows strangers to sell an organ and leaves would-be recipients in the position of having to choose between law and life. More, when giving something as singular as an organ, a donor is unlikely to feel that "he comes today and is gone tomorrow." All gifts carry an expectation of reciprocity, whether articulated or not. This dynamic resonates even more deeply when it comes to a body part. The question is not whether there will be an expectation (and reality) of reciprocity, but what specific form the reciprocity will take. The donor may expect or demand monetary compensation, and the grateful recipient may feel obliged to agree.

Third, to the extent that Internet use encourages donations from strangers, it increases the risk of unacceptable harm. The risk-benefit ratio changes markedly when a stranger's bodily integrity is at stake. From the time that the first kidney transplant occurred between twins, courts and commentators have upheld the idea that the benefits to a sibling for having kept alive his twin far outweighed the risks of living with one kidney.[28] But this calculation does not extend to strangers. Even if the risk of the procedure and its long-term consequences are low, it is difficult to identify what offsetting benefit to the donor has been served.

Fourth, the digital divide between those with Internet access and those without raises concerns about the potential for the Web to exacerbate already existing inequities within the field of transplantation. In 1995, a government report "Falling Through the Net" described the digital divide to be one of "America's leading economic and civil rights issues."[29] While access to the Internet has expanded, there still remain a high number of people who lack such access. According to the Pew Report, "Digital Divisions," one-third of American adults, or about 65 million people, do not use the Internet. The report also notes that lack of access is "not always by choice." Socio-economic factors, such as age, race, and education, are associated with Internet access: only 26 percent of Americans age sixty-five years or older go online, compared with

67 percent of those age fifty to sixty-four, 80 percent of those thirty to forty-nine, and 84 percent of those age eighteen to twenty-nine. While 70 percent of whites go online, the proportion for African Americans is 57 percent. Finally, those without a high school diploma go online significantly less (29 percent) than those with high school diplomas (61 percent) and college degrees (89 percent).[30]

Policy Challenges

Given both the potential advantages and disadvantages of online organ procurement, the transplant community has not been able to formulate a consistent response to Web donors. The United Network for Organ Sharing (UNOS), the leading American transplant organization and government contractor responsible for setting national policy on organ transplantation, initially aligned itself with the opposition camp. In June 2004, UNOS resolved to "philosophically oppose the program being marketed by matchingdonors.com, as it exploits vulnerable populations and undermines public trust in the equitable allocation of organs for transplant."[31] Shortly thereafter, however, UNOS moved from resistance to resignation and then on to acceptance. As UNOS President and transplant surgeon, Francis Delmonico, observed: "I don't think we can legislate or regulate how people get to know each other. . . . Once that occurs and someone decides they want to save another person, I don't think we ought to stop that as long as they are medically suitable, are not violating the law and are fully informed."[32]

In addition to being unable to discourage the practice, UNOS had difficulty regulating it. Attempts to create standard guidelines for accepting living donors, let alone Web donors, have met with dogged resistance from transplant teams. They insisted that any effort at standardization of practice infringed upon their autonomy to decide what was best for their patients and what donors to accept. Each transplant center follows its own acceptance criteria for living organ donors and sets its own "philosophy for providing live donor transplantation." They have no intention of giving up any of their prerogatives. Because there is extraordinary variation in practice among transplant teams, ranging from teams "accepting only known relatives or those with close emotional ties to those approving transplants from non-directed donors or those with only distant relationships," consensus on Web donation could not be achieved.[33]

Transplant centers themselves continue to be divided over online organ solicitation. In a recent survey on the willingness of transplant centers to consider an "Internet-identified live kidney donor" for a transplant patient, 37 percent (76 of the 206 U.S. kidney transplant centers) indicated a willingness to accept such a donor. When queried further, all 76 centers stated that the donor would have to undergo the medical team's evaluation, including medical and psychosocial assessments. Each of these centers also emphasized that financial exchange for an organ was illegal. Eight of them also acknowledged that they had already performed such Internet-based transplants and would be willing to do so again.[34] In all, transplant teams continue to respond to Web donors on a case by case basis, to resist setting a common policy, and to avoid coming to terms with the full meaning of the Internet for the medical profession and society at large.

Implications for the Medical Professional

Following on the Madison and Hall chapter, let us conclude by placing the issues of information technology and organ donation directly into the context of professionalism. Using the American Board of Internal Medicine's Physician Charter on professionalism as our guidepost,[35] we are specifically concerned with the relevance of our findings on kidney donation to its three core principles: patient welfare, patient autonomy, and social justice.

The Primacy of Patients' Welfare

Advocates for Internet solicitation for organs argue that their position represents the best interest of patients. Whatever the possible adverse social consequences, the patient receives an organ in a more timely manner and thereby reaps considerable health benefits. Advocates also contend that online solicitation increases the supply of organs, benefiting all ESRD patients. These donations add more organs to the pool, and thereby, reduce shortfall. Not only does one fortunate patient have an organ but all those below him or her on the waiting list move up one slot.

These contentions, however, are not persuasive. The principle of patient welfare was never intended to justify any or all behavior, unethical as well as illegal, which might work to the benefit of a particular patient. Further, the effect of these donations is less "trickle down" and more "skimming the bottom." The solicited organ often alleviates a shortage among patients who are of low priority—they are new to the wait list and generally in much better health. Those in greatest need of an organ remain at the top of the list, with no accrued benefit from the donation.

Patient Autonomy

Advocates of online solicitation of organs argue that physician respect for patient autonomy should encourage transplant teams to approve donor-patient matches facilitated by the Web. Not to do so is to behave in a highly paternalistic fashion. As one transplant team leader insisted: "To assume that we control everything and so we get to decide and everyone else is going to accept our judgment because we are the doctors is to fall prey to an arrogance that is just not a luxury we have."[36] Medicine, therefore, should not proscribe strangers from performing altruistic acts—telling individuals what they may or may not do. Indeed, by objecting to donations solicited from strangers, teams may be blocking upward mobility for the poor, at least to the degree that some unknown and unknowable percentage of these "donations" will bring donors clandestine payments. Since directed donation is considered safe enough for families and friends, why discriminate against strangers, even financially motivated strangers?

Critics insist that such arguments misconstrue the principle of patient autonomy. It is not a rule that sanctions all behaviors, including the harmful and illegal. Patient preferences should carry great weight but they are not absolute. A physician's deference to a patient's choice cannot be at odds with "ethical practice" and "appropriate care." Patient autonomy does not justify a physician responding to a demand by prescribing the wrong drug, performing an unnecessary operation, or in this instance, ignoring the history of the organ in the freezer chest. Teams must not become accomplices to immoral and illegal acts.

Social Justice

The principle of social justice offers the most clear-cut rationale for rejecting Web-based organ solicitation. Web sites such as matchingdonors.com not only discriminate against those with fewer resources but also promote values that should not be determinative of the distribution of medical resources. Advocates of the Web argue that organ transplantation, like so many other medical procedures, from biopsies to bypasses, favors patients with greater social and economic assets. Why then single out the Web? Why permit living organ donation but exercise caution over online solicitation? What makes Web donors any different? The answer rests in the fact that online solicitation makes medical practice complicit with an inappropriate allocation system. The very practice of seeking out strangers online for an organ not only promotes greater inequality in access to care but also patently discriminatory practices. When we move from the confines of friends and family into the world of strangers, we shift from the private to the public realm. And social values that are appropriate and powerful within a private context should not hold sway in a public context.

The most infamous example of how private sentiment cannot be allowed to determine public medical practice is the case of a Florida man who became brain-dead and who had earlier consented to donate his organs. Both the man and his family set one condition for the donation: the organ recipient had to be white. Although the transplant team honored the request, an uproar over the stipulation ensued, and the state soon enacted a law barring patients or families from using personal prejudice to restrict donations.[37] Medical practice should not be bound by racist prejudices.

While not as egregious as the whites-only condition, online solicitation ultimately allows social worth, a category once deemed unacceptable in the allocation of medical resources, to regain prominence. Now, as in the Seattle dialysis days, the bachelor is out of the running, and so are the unemployed, the childless, and the atheists. You may not want to date such a person, or have him or her adopt your child. That is a private choice. But to approve a public system of recruitment that promotes the importance of such discriminations in medical practice is not consistent with the values of medical professionalism. The core principles are not as novel as the Internet technology, but that does not make them any less potent or relevant.

Changing the Rules

The Impact of Information Technology on Contemporary Maternity Practice

I now make my last appeal to every woman who has read this book to take up the battle for painless childbirth where I have left off. . . . Fight not only for yourselves, but fight for your sister-mothers, your sex, the cradle of the human race. Realize . . . the tremendous importance . . . of removing the dread of birth pain from the mind of women, a dread which has steadily grown until it has developed into a social menace."

Hannah Rion[1]

I think that [cesarean] is . . . the best way . . . to give birth. It is a planned way, no hassle, no pain, the baby doesn't struggle to come out, the baby is not pressed to come out. . . . I think that . . . everybody should have the baby by cesarean section."

Anonymous respondent to national survey in 2006[2]

Each of these quotes written a century apart identifies an intervention that will redress the pain of childbirth. The absolute faith in a technological innovation is a central theme in American medicine. In the case of maternity care practice, information technology has played a less obvious role than in other fields of medicine, however, it was a critical component of the campaign of obstetricians to gain control of maternity care practice in the twentieth century. As the twenty-first century begins, however, the development of multiple specialized sources of information on pregnancy and childbirth is providing mothers with the foundation to challenge that hard-won control. The story begins a century ago.

As the twentieth century began, the challenge faced by male doctors in the emerging specialty of obstetrics was a simple one—how could physicians develop a respected medical specialty when the same work they proposed to do was being carried out by female midwives, many with limited training. Equally frustrating to physicians, the outcomes of midwife-attended births were usually better than the results of physician-attended births, since midwives were generally far more experienced birth attendants.[3] Most European countries solved this problem by restructuring practice and developing screening protocols to identify lower risk births which would be attended by midwives while obstetricians became specialists in managing high-risk cases.[4] In the United States (and Canada and South Africa) the goal was different—to eliminate midwifery with obstetricians taking control of low- as well as high-risk births.

The key to achieving this goal was information technology (IT), not as a unified concept but in terms of controlling the use of information and technology to further obstetrics. Information was conveyed by contemporary media (primarily advice books and women's and popular magazines) to redefine birth as a dangerous event.[5] Technology was critical to the claim that only those in control of the latest, most sophisticated systems could protect mothers and infants from the deadly outcomes associated with birth. Of additional importance to many women, innovations such as Twilight Sleep were being touted as rendering childbirth painless.[6]

Twilight Sleep, at that time a mixture of scopolamine and morphine, was not an anesthetic but an amnesiac causing a woman to have little or no memory of her childbirth experience. Developed in Germany in the early twentieth century it soon became popular in the United States.[7] Since Twilight Sleep could only be administered by a physician in a hospital, its use significantly shifted not only the domain of birth away from the female-controlled home to the male-dominated hospital, but, since midwives were denied hospital privileges, altered who could attend births in the United States.

Equally important, this new technology became tied to an information campaign that focused on doctors as the most reliable source of information on pregnancy and childbirth. In essence, the nascent profession of obstetrics took advantage of the opportunity provided by new media (books and magazines) to lay the foundation for control of the flow of information concerning pregnancy and birth. The burgeoning women's movements at the time were critical to this effort, leading to the formation of Twilight Sleep Societies advocating for more widespread use of the new drugs. These campaigns emphasized the frailty of "refined" women and the need to protect them from the scourge of pain in childbirth.[8]

The results of these efforts powerfully supported the redefinition of birth from being a natural event to one that was so fraught with danger that only a trained doctor in a hospital with the latest technology could prevent disastrous outcomes. In this case, a technological innovation combined with an information campaign to reshape maternal perspectives on childbirth, foster the elevation of the hospital as the center of scientific and technological intervention, and promote the obstetrician as the safest option for birthing mothers. This trend continued throughout the twentieth century as birth became increasingly organized to address the needs of institutions, providers, and the new technologies that enhanced obstetricians' control of the process.[9]

IT and Contemporary Maternity Care Providers

Birth is unlike any other area of medicine since it involves the management of a condition of health rather than sickness. The process of pregnancy and childbirth is largely predictable and in most cases, if medical personnel played no role whatsoever, mother and baby would still be fine. This substantially changes the nature of clinical decision-making from typically trying to diagnose the source of an illness or treating an already diagnosed illness to attempting to predict who among a healthy population may develop a condition that would put a woman or her baby at risk. The need to protect the health of two conjoined patients at once simply added to the complexity of the decision-making involved.

Both changes internal to the practice of maternity care and the profession of obstetrics and external ones in the increasing access of mothers to information on their experiences have shaped the recent history of information technology in maternity care. After a brief review of these changes, this chapter will turn to the current challenge faced by the profession of obstetrics—the proliferation of information sources only partly or not at all controlled by obstetrical providers.

Information Technology and Contemporary
Maternity Care Decision Making

The past three decades have seen an explosion of scientific knowledge about the birth process. There has also been a concomitant rise in the promise of information technology to provide more and better information to aid in clinical decision-making with the application of models to sort out the increasing flow of information. The American College of Obstetricians and Gynecologists (ACOG) took the lead in the late 1980s to establish an integrated academic information management system (IAIMS) termed ACOGQUEST for the profession with great promise for improving clinical care.[10] It was the only professional organization to receive a grant from the National Library of Medicine for this purpose (ten academic centers also received grants) and the College's goal focused on four areas: member educational programs on information technology, development of a prototype OB-GYN knowledge base, improvement of membership services, and integration with other IAIMS systems.[11] Despite this initiative, physician practice studies have suggested that obstetricians appear to be somewhat late adopters of new information technology, being significantly less likely than other physicians to utilize IT to access patient notes and exchange information with other physicians or with hospitals.[12]

Recent discussions in the obstetrics literature have been more muted about the role of information technology (the ACOGQUEST project did not receive implementation funding from the NIH). In his 2005 ACOG presidential address, Michael Mennuti cited the need for the profession to respond to broader changes, specifically the increasing importance of genomic medicine and information technology. His comments concerning IT emphasized the benefits to "performance evaluation to track productivity, efficiency and quality of care,"[13] as well as training. He also noted the challenge IT represented to medical liability with more detailed permanent written records, as opposed to telephone or personal conversations (see chapter 4 in this book for additional examples). He made this point more forcefully in testifying before Congress in 2005 when he called for information collected by government funders to be exempt from medical liability or in hiring and retention cases.[14] Two specific applications of information technology in maternity care illustrate its potential and its limitations for impacting practice: the evidence-based medicine movement and the use of electronic fetal monitoring.

Evidence-based obstetrics

In 1979, physician and epidemiologist Archie Cochrane awarded obstetrics his "wooden spoon" award for the specialty of medicine that was the least evidence based. A decade later, writing the foreword to the book *Effective Care in Pregnancy and Childbirth*, he withdrew that insult claiming that the publication of *Effective Care* signaled a new day in obstetric practice.[15] In essence, the specialty of medicine deemed the least evidence based had begun to lead the way in developing a model for systematically documenting and disseminating the results of randomized trials in all areas of medicine. Of particular interest was the compilation and dissemination by the National Perinatal Epidemiology Unit (NPEU) at Oxford in Britain of the results of hundreds of randomized trials in maternity care.

Of course, systematically compiling evidence on best practices does not ensure those practices will be implemented and, in maternity care, the results have been mixed. In some areas, (folic acid supplementation, use of vacuum extraction over forceps, use of prophylactic antibiotics prior to a cesarean, reductions in the use of enemas and perineal shaving) the results of trials or meta-analyses have been largely adopted in practice. In other areas, such as fetal monitoring and the use of episiotomies, the results of clinical trials have had limited or no impact on practice.

As information from randomized clinical trials and other systematic studies grew rapidly, the challenge for clinicians became how to keep up with and assess the applicability of the flood of information they were facing and the new technologies promised to help. As far back as 1979, Iain Chalmers, founder of the NPEU, had written a meta-analysis of published trials in obstetrical practice summarizing their results for clinicians.[16] These became a regular feature of the work of the NPEU and later the Cochrane Collaboration, a center for the development and publication of systematic reviews of the effects of healthcare interventions, and are now a routine component of the medical literature. The problem has become one of sorting through the dizzying array of new findings to determine their significance and relevance to clinical decision-making. Ironically, one major effort to synthesize research findings for obstetricians appears not to have utilized the Cochrane evidence-based reviews. A 2008 study examined the "Clinical Expert Series" in the journal *Obstetrics & Gynecology*—the official publication of the American College of Obstetricians and Gynecologists. Of the fifty-four articles in the series since its inception, there were references to Cochrane reviews in only nineteen of thirty-six cases where such reviews were published at least two years prior to the expert series articles.[17]

Also currently assisting clinicians is the development of a number of clinical information brokers who, often with electronic newsletter formats (see, for example, www.medscape.com), sort through published studies and provide synopses of materials for clinicians too busy to read or unable to understand the statistical methods of articles in the myriad journals with findings on obstetrics. The leaders of the profession have also taken on this responsibility with the American College of Obstetricians and Gynecologists providing a comparable service with the above mentioned "Clinical Expert series." In essence the rise in information available to clinicians is driving the development of new information technology tools to help them deal with sorting through and contextualizing evidence.

Electronic fetal monitoring

Electronic fetal monitoring (EFM) emerged with great promise in the late 1960s. It appeared that continuously recording both the baby's heartbeat and the strength of a mother's contraction would provide crucial information to identify infants at risk and allow timely interventions to prevent, for example, cerebral palsy. The difficulty was that study after study came up with similar findings—fetal monitoring of women already identified as high risk was valuable, but for the large majority of women otherwise not at risk it provided no benefit and was linked to higher rates of unnecessary interventions.[18] Nonetheless, despite consistent findings of its limited value, often in articles with titles such as "Paradox of Fetal Monitoring,"[19] "Uncertain Value of EFM,"[20] and a review article in 2000 titled, "Fetal Heart Rate Monitoring: Is It Salvageable?"[21] the use of EFM is virtually universal.[22] In the case of EFM, the lure of a promising new information technology aimed at assisting clinical decision-making led to the universal adoption of the technology by clinicians despite its failure to provide a significant benefit for most patients. This represents one of the important difficulties in the growing use of IT—the adoption of technologies largely for the symbolic value they represent as advancing practice.

The impact of changes in models of practice on
the role of obstetricians as information sources

Also shaping the role of information technology on maternity care practices has been shifts in the nature of obstetrical practice that have impacted the role of obstetricians as filters of information on maternity care.[23] These changes have included the challenging malpractice environment, constraints on reimbursement, and a desire by obstetricians for a better lifestyle. One response to this changing climate has been the rise in group practices. Group practices, long a common feature of many specialties, represented a major shift in the model of obstetrical practice. A crucial element in the development of the attachment between obstetricians and their patients was the extraordinary commitment made by individual obstetricians—that they would attend the mother in labor regardless of day of week or time of day. This commitment engendered enormous trust among patients, but made for bad working conditions for obstetricians who might have to visit a hospital several times to check in on mothers in labor while rushing back to the office to manage care for other patients. An obvious solution was the development of group practices with clearer hours for office and on-call periods.[24] One national study estimated that 39 percent of obstetricians were in solo or two-physician practices in 2004–2005, slightly above the national average for all physicians.[25] The natural extension of this shift has been the proposal of a new model of care based on the hospitalist, in this case a "laborist," who would be a hospital-based obstetrician attending deliveries while community-based obstetricians would focus on prenatal, postpartum and gynecological care.[26] These models make considerable sense to obstetricians and provide an opportunity for continuity of care (but not of care provider) in a model common in European countries, but further sever the personal ties that previously made U.S. obstetricians such a prime source of information for mothers. At the same time, physicians are under pressure from funders to maintain short visits, with an average visit to an obstetrician-gynecologist lasting just seventeen minutes in 2004.[27] As David Blumenthal points out (chapter 1 in this book), health information technology has the potential to improve or hinder the doctor-patient relationship, but in any case it will significantly alter it and those changes have already begun to be manifested in obstetrics.

The decreasing connection of obstetricians with patients continues in labor with 19 percent of mothers in a national survey saying that they never met the person who delivered their baby and another 9 percent saying they had only briefly met that individual.[28] An obstetrician's contact with mothers in labor is also lessened by the rise of a new subspecialty—the obstetrical anesthesiologist. In the past obstetricians were crucial to mothers in labor since they were the source of medications that provided pain relief, but now even that role has been supplanted with the advent of epidurals which are typically administered by specially trained anesthesiologists. With three-fourths of all U.S. mothers (76 percent) now receiving epidurals[29] the obstetrical-anesthesiologist has become the most significant clinician for many mothers during labor. Finally the rise in malpractice suits can be seen as both a cause and a result of the deteriorating relationship between mothers and obstetricians, further undermining the role of the obstetrician as the source of critical information for the mother. Obstetricians now have to be increasingly careful in framing what they say to mothers for fear it will become evidence in a later lawsuit and, as noted above, the use of written responses (e.g., in e-mails) to questions has been a matter of concern for the creation of evidence to be used in a potential lawsuit. This climate is not lost on mothers, 42 percent of who in a national survey agreed with the statement that obstetricians sometimes performed unnecessary cesareans in order to avoid a lawsuit.[30] The result of these changes is seen below, where first-time mothers did not rank their doctors as their primary source of information on pregnancy and childbirth. We now explore the alternatives to which consumers have turned.

The Changing Nature of Consumer Decision-Making in Maternity Care

Research on the impact of alternative information sources on health has emphasized the continued primacy of physicians as trusted sources of health information in general.[31] However, these and other studies document growing use of alternative sources.[32] In the case of maternity care, historically there was a reliance on family, friends, and local midwives for advice. In time, male physicians, first as family doctors and later as obstetricians, began to play a more significant role in the provision of information. The development of prenatal care, a twentieth-century phenomenon, helped formalize the status of the doctor as a source of information. Critical to this elevation of the physician was the redefinition of birth as something other than a normal event.[33] The more dangerous birth appeared to be, the more necessary it was for it to occur in a hospital (an institution also being redefined as a center of science at that time) under the supervision of a physician.

As literacy expanded and books became inexpensive to produce, advice manuals on pregnancy and birth (and almost every other health condition) also became popular. These advice manuals generally focused on natural or homeopathic remedies,[34] and a component of the professionalization of obstetrics was to move mothers to more scientific approaches to managing pregnancy and childbirth. The goal was to establish obstetricians as the prime and, ideally, the only source of wisdom on appropriate maternity care. The extraordinary time commitment obstetricians made to mothers and families described above further cemented strong and long-lasting relationships to women.

The success of that campaign led to the increasing dominance of male obstetricians over the birthing process, abetted by the development of drugs like Twilight Sleep, a legal campaign against midwives,[35] and ultimately the hospitalization of virtually all births by the early 1940s.[36] This dominance eventually led to a backlash starting in the 1950s. Some mothers rebelled against the idea of being heavily drugged during childbirth. The perceived great benefit of Twilight Sleep—the ability of the drugs to eliminate or blur the memory of the birth experience—became precisely the concern of mothers who wanted to be more in control of the birthing process.[37] Both the titles and content of popular books at the time, such as *Awake and Aware*,[38] *Childbirth without Fear*,[39] and *Thank You Dr. Lamaze*,[40] challenged physician dominance over the flow of information (though ironically the first two books were written by doctors) about childbirth.

A more direct challenge took the form of the establishment of childbirth education classes, which were associated with what was termed the natural childbirth movement. These classes relied on independent, home-based female childbirth educators who focused on both preparation for birth and female empowerment.[41] As these classes became increasingly popular in the 1970s, efforts to co-opt these classes began.[42] The co-optation was in the form of moving classes from educators' homes to hospitals and doctors' offices where they could now serve a two-fold purpose. They were used in advertising campaigns as marketing tools for institutions seeking new patients and the content of the classes could be better controlled by those institutions. The success of those efforts can be seen in the institutionalization of classes with almost nine out of ten childbirth classes now taught in hospitals or doctors' offices, by employees of those institutions. These changes altered the focus of classes from empowering women to make decisions for themselves to an emphasis on preparing mothers for the birth experience they could expect with their doctor's practice in a particular hospital. These efforts apparently succeeded, with a national survey of mothers who gave birth in 2005 finding those attending classes eleven times more likely to agree than disagree that the classes helped them communicate better with their providers, eight times more likely to report greater trust in their providers, seven times more likely to report having greater trust in their birthing hospitals, and three times as likely to report less fear of interventions.[43]

Contemporary Challenges to Physician Control of Information Sources

Just as the rise in literacy in the early twentieth century spawned new advice books on pregnancy and childbirth, the rise of new media at the outset of the twenty-first century contains a challenge to and an opportunity for physicians to control the information process. Two new media in particular—the Internet and specialized cable television—present unique tests for physicians' control of the information process. In both instances obstetricians have played a role in the development of content for the media and, in both cases, the media have generally maintained some independence from physician control. There is an obvious desire for obstetrician input to enhance the credibility of these media, but the desire for independence is less a matter of philosophical disagreement with obstetricians and more a function of the intent to structure content to appeal to the most profitable audience (either as a result of total audience size or targeted market segment) possible.

Evidence for the importance of new information sources in health care in general and maternity care in particular is seen in a variety of studies. The Pew Internet and American Life Project has done a series of national surveys on Internet use and has found increasing levels of use of the Internet for searching for health information. While men (76 percent) and women (74 percent) reported similar rates of usage, women were more likely (81 percent to 66 percent) to use the Internet to seek health information;[44] confidence in the reliability of Internet sources was increasing among users;[45] and the surveys document the oft noted "digital divide,"[46] with minorities and lower income individuals less likely to have Internet access.[47] Blacks and Hispanics were less likely to have

Table 7.1   **Most Important Information Source for Mothers, by Parity**

While pregnant, most important source of information about being pregnant and giving birth	First-time mothers (n = 444) %	Experienced mothers (n = 927) %
Books	33	12
Friends and/or relatives	19	7
Internet	16	13
Doctor	14	16
Childbirth education class	10	1
Midwife	4	2
Mass media	2	1
Own experiences from a previous labor and birth	0	48
Other	2	1

Source: Adapted from E. R. Declercq, C. Sakala, M. P. Corry, and S. Applebaum, *Listening to Mothers II: Report of the Second National U.S. Survey of Women's Childbearing Experiences* (New York: Childbirth Connection, 2006).

*p < .01 for difference between mothers by prior birth experience

Internet access, although what is interesting is that among those who did, English-speaking Latinos reported rates of usage comparable to or higher than white non-Hispanics.[48] Overall 79 percent of Internet users reported that they searched online for health information in areas such as diet, fitness, and drug information.[49] Less is known about Internet use concerning pregnancy and childbirth, though a small Canadian study of attendees at prenatal classes found almost 50 percent of the mothers reporting they used the Internet as a source "a lot" and 50 percent saying they used it "some."[50]

The Listening to Mothers II survey of 1573 U.S. mothers (see appendix to this chapter for a summary of the survey methods) included a series of questions concerning prenatal information sources and we include those results here. In table 7.1 the data are stratified by whether or not a mother was giving birth for the first time or had given birth before. Clearly, in the latter case, mothers were most likely to rely on their own past experiences, followed by their doctor, the Internet, and books as their primary information sources. Of greater interest is where new mothers acquire their information on pregnancy and birth. Perhaps surprisingly, the highest ranked information source was books (33 percent), followed by friends or relatives (19 percent), and the Internet (16 percent). The high ranking of books is not surprising when one looks at the

Table 7.2   **Most Important Information Source for First-Time Mothers by Race/Ethnicity**

While pregnant, most important source of information about being pregnant and giving birth	% White non-Hispanic (n = 325)	% Black non-Hispanic (n = 42)	% Hispanic (n = 56)
Books	35	36	13
Friends and/or relatives	18	10	34
Internet	15	14	20
Doctor	16	10	7
Childbirth education class	8	19	13
Midwife	4	0	11
Mass media	2	0	4

Source: Adapted from E. R. Declercq, C. Sakala, M. P. Corry, and S. Applebaum, *Listening to Mothers II: Report of the Second National U.S. Survey of Women's Childbearing Experiences* (New York: Childbirth Connection, 2006).

*p < .01 for difference between mothers by race/ethnicity

sales figures of the most popular guide for expectant mothers, *What to Expect When You're Expecting*,[51] which has sold 14 million copies and was still ranked third on the *New York Times* advice bestseller list in 2008, more than two decades after it was initially published. The success of *What to Expect*, which has spawned a cottage industry of related books and products, has been a result of the ongoing interest in advice books, a great title, and a conservative, doctor-compatible view of birth that has generated heated criticism from women's groups.[52]

The two information sources most directly controlled by physicians (doctors themselves and childbirth classes) accounted for 24 percent of first-time mothers and only 17 percent of experienced mothers' primary sources of information. Doctors themselves only ranked fourth as sources among new mothers. The mass media was not rated as among mothers' primary sources of information, though some specific sources were relied on as will be evident below. Different patterns emerge when first-time mothers are stratified by race/ethnicity in table 7.2 with 54 percent of Hispanic mothers being most likely to rely on either friends, relatives, or the Internet for information compared to 33 percent for whites and 24 percent for blacks. Black mothers relied most commonly on books (36 percent) and childbirth classes (19 percent) while, for white mothers, books (35 percent) led the way. As a primary source of information on pregnancy and birth, doctors were rated third by white non-Hispanic mothers (16 percent), fourth by black non-Hispanic mothers, and sixth (7 percent) by Hispanic mothers.

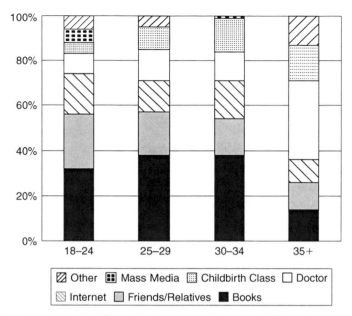

Figure 7.1 First-Time Mothers' Most Important Sources of Information on Pregnancy and Birth, by Age (n = 471)

Source: Adapted from E. R. Declercq, C. Sakala, M. P. Corry, and S. Applebaum, *Listening to Mothers II: Report of the Second National U.S. Survey of Women's Childbearing Experiences* (New York: Childbirth Connection, 2006).

There is one demographic group for which doctors retain their authoritative role and that is among older mothers (figure 7.1). First-time mothers over age thirty-five rated doctors as their most important source of information (37 percent) on pregnancy and birth—a rate three times that of mothers in any other age group. This may be a result of older first-time mothers facing more difficult births and whose pregnancies may have involved assisted reproductive technologies (ART), since 20 percent of mothers thirty-five and older relied on ART in becoming pregnant.[53] The survey also found that a large proportion of mothers agreed with the position long held by physicians that birth is a medical, rather than a normal physiological event. Only 50 percent of mothers agreed with the statement, "Birth is a process that should not be interfered with unless medically necessary,"[54] and not surprisingly, mothers thirty-five and older were the least likely to agree with that statement.

Role of the Internet

One in six (16 percent) first-time mothers and 13 percent of experienced mothers cited the Internet as their main source of information on pregnancy and birth. The "digital divide" was not as apparent in terms of race/ethnicity with

Hispanic mothers (20 percent) most likely to cite the Internet as their primary source. This finding is consistent with other research on Internet usage for other health information finding that English-speaking Hispanics (the Listening to Mothers II survey was available only in English) were heavy users of the Internet.[55] Obstetricians anecdotally cite mothers' use of the Internet in asking questions about the nature of their maternity care, though there is little direct research on the phenomenon.[56]

Mothers' reliance on the Internet as their primary data source was not surprisingly related to age (figure 7.1), with mothers aged eighteen to twenty-four slightly more likely to cite the Internet as their most important source, and with mothers aged thirty-five and older least likely. Mothers, regardless of whether or not they cited the Internet as their primary source of information, were asked if they *ever* used the Internet to gather information on pregnancy and childbirth and 73 percent had done so. White mothers (79 percent) were most likely to have used the Internet to gather such information. Mothers who did use the Internet reported a median of forty-five visits during their pregnancy with mothers aged twenty-five to twenty-nine (average of fifty-two visits) the most frequent users.

Role of mass media as an information source
The marketing potential of reaching 4 million new parents a year in a targeted way has provided the financial and infrastructure support to develop a number of new initiatives to shape the flow of information to mothers. In the case of mass media, television, with its plethora of specialized channels can now devote an inordinate amount of attention to the particular question of childbirth. While mothers rarely cited the media as their primary source of information, there have been at least eight shows devoted to childbirth that have been in regular rotation on cable networks. Fully 68 percent of mothers reported viewing at least one of these shows—significantly more mothers than reported attending a childbirth class (25 percent).[57]

One show ("A Baby Story") was reportedly viewed regularly by almost one-third of all mothers in the survey—a finding made more plausible by the fact that the show was broadcast up to four times a day on the Learning Channel. It completed its tenth season in 2008 and has broadcast more than 500 different "stories" since its premiere. Two other shows, "Birth Day" and "Babies: Special Delivery" (both aired on Discovery Health) also were regularly viewed by at least 20 percent of mothers. First-time mothers in particular (78 percent) reported watching these shows. The results presented in table 7.3 suggest that watching the shows had an impact since more than seven out of ten

Table 7.3   **Impact of TV Shows Dedicated to Birth on First-Time
Mothers**

What impact did the program have on you as a pregnant woman?	%
Helped me understand what it would be like to give birth	72
Helped me feel excited about upcoming birth	59
Helped me learn about medical words and technology	48
Helped me clarify my preferences for birth	38
Caused me to worry about my upcoming birth	32

Source: Adapted from E. R. Declercq, C. Sakala, M. P. Corry, and S. Applebaum,
*Listening to Mothers II: Report of the Second National U.S. Survey of Women's
Childbearing Experiences* (New York: Childbirth Connection, 2006).
Base: (p) Watched TV shows on birth (n = 272)

first-time mothers (72 percent) reported that the shows helped them understand what the process of birth would be like and three in five (59 percent)
agreed that the shows made them more excited about birth. Notably, one in
three first-time mothers (32 percent) said the shows caused them to become
more worried about their upcoming birth. As one respondent noted in her
open-ended comments, "[Birth] was a wonderful experience. It was not at all as
painful and dramatic as they show on TV during "Maternity Ward" or things
like that. . . . I did not do all that screaming."

Changing the Rules

What is the impact of these new sources of information on obstetrics as a profession? Research on one key aspect of this question—doctor-patient relations—
has been focused on patient surveys that ask both about the use of other
information sources (primarily the Internet) and about how patients rated their
doctor's response to their use of that information. Elizabeth Murray in a nationally representative telephone survey of patients found 31 percent of respondents had used the Internet for health information in the past year.[58] Those
respondents indicated several possible difficulties that could arise from the
Internet information including unnecessary visits to a physician, taking up
more of a physician's time, and the possibility that it would interfere with the
doctor-patient relationship. They found few respondents (4 percent) had
scheduled a specific visit to ask about information gathered from the Internet,
with most just raising issues in an already scheduled visit. When patients
brought questions to their physicians, it was generally to ask their opinion about
the information they had discovered.

Respondents reported that physicians reacted positively (67 percent) or neutrally (27 percent) to the information with only 7 percent citing a negative reaction. However, 15 percent also indicated that their physician had "acted challenged" by the information. Only 4 percent reported they thought the information had harmed their relationship with their doctor. Factors perceived by the patients that were related to the likelihood of a poorer relationship with their doctor included the degree to which the doctor acted challenged by the information, the doctor's communication skills, or if the patient felt hurried during the visit. A similar study of men with prostate cancer bringing Internet based information to their doctors had generally comparable findings with the doctor's communication skills being seen as the key element in how the information was received. One respondent indicated that his doctor took his list of questions and simply replied "yes, no, yes, no, not applicable, yes, no."[59]

The evolution of sources of information in maternity care—from midwives and women family members to advice books and doctors to childbirth classes and now the Internet and specialized television shows has impacted the authoritative position obstetricians once occupied as the primary source of information concerning childbirth. Some of this has been the result of changes in the nature of obstetrical practice. From sole practitioners attending mothers in labor at all hours, the profession has changed to group practices with short visits, obstetrical anesthesiologists being the source of pain relief, and a mother having almost a one in three chance of barely having met the doctor who delivered her baby.

While mothers have always had alternative sources of information on pregnancy and childbirth, for a time in the 1980s and 1990s it seemed as if doctors had the best of both worlds—they retained their authoritative status as providers of information and they had considerable control over the other major source of information, childbirth education classes. Childbirth education classes continue to be held in hospitals or doctors' offices, but far fewer mothers now attend them and obstetricians face new challenges to their control of the flow of information. They have responded with initiatives aimed at retaining that control with the American College of Obstetricians and Gynecologists setting up a consumer-friendly portion of its Web site and acting as a major source for distribution of educational materials. There are also significant attempts to continue to redefine birth as a medical procedure with a new genre of literature developing on the dangers of vaginal birth.[60]

As the other chapters in this volume point out, significant attempts have been made to provide greater access to health information by both doctors and patients. However the increase in the flow of information has been so overwhelming that it has buried all parties in data and the new challenge is sorting out the significant from the dross. This chapter has presented a case study of how the profession of obstetrics has dealt with this challenge. The past century has seen the rise of the obstetrician as the authoritative figure in controlling the flow of information to mothers and part of the obstetricians' professional success has been in adapting to new forms of information technology to stay ahead of their patients. There is little reason to expect that adaptability not to continue, but the democratizing of the flow of health information may be the most significant challenge yet for obstetricians.

Appendix: *Listening to Mothers II* Methodology

The Listening to Mothers II survey was developed through collaborative efforts of core teams from Childbirth Connection, the Boston University School of Public Health, and Harris Interactive®, with the support of the Listening to Mothers II National Advisory Council and in partnership with Lamaze International. Harris Interactive administered the survey. For Listening to Mothers II, 200 mothers were interviewed by telephone, and 1,373 completed an online version of the survey. All 1,573 survey participants had given birth to a single baby (mothers with multiple births were excluded) in a hospital in 2005. The interviews, averaging approximately thirty minutes in length, were conducted in January–February 2006.

There were many indications that the mothers were exceptionally engaged in the survey and interested in having their voices heard, including their willingness to take more time answering questions than typical survey respondents and to provide detailed responses to open-ended questions that asked about best and worst aspects of their experiences while giving birth. The researchers made special efforts to ensure a representative national sample through the over-sampling of mothers who were ethnic minorities in the telephone portion of the survey. To develop a national profile of childbearing women, the data were adjusted with demographic and propensity score weightings using methodology developed and validated by Harris Interactive. The resulting survey population is representative of U.S. mothers aged eighteen to forty-five who gave birth to a single infant in a hospital in 2005. The respondents are generally comparable to those in published national data for U.S. birthing mothers on critical factors such as age, race/ethnicity, parity, birth attendant, and method of birth. A total of 903 of the original mothers participated in the postpartum survey, either online or by phone, in July–August 2006, and those data were likewise weighted to obtain a nationally representative view of the target population.

The questions on sources of information about pregnancy, use of the Internet and all demographic characteristics were drawn from the original survey. The question on watching of television shows was included in the postpartum survey. For a more complete report on the survey methodology, see the *Listening to Mothers II* report and/or an article that details the methods (2) (from the Listening to Mothers II report).

A Profession of IT's Own

The Rise of Health Information Professionals in American Health Care

Professionalism means many things to many people, and those meanings are sometimes at odds with one another. In some accounts, professionalism means simply the ethical and competent practice of a particular set of occupational skills. Other accounts add a dispositional component, such as a lifelong commitment to client service, or to the mastery and embellishment of a particular body of knowledge. And still other (often darker) views emphasize political and economic dimensions, such as the capacity to control entry into, and practice within, a lucrative market niche, or the ability to assert authority and command deference in the workplace.

An expanded reliance on new information technologies will undoubtedly affect all these aspects of professionalism in the medical arena. As clinical information technology (IT) grows in prevalence and power, medical professionals will increasingly interact with patients through digital media, make care decisions in light of computerized data, and perform medical procedures by electronic control, sometimes over great distances and across multiple legal jurisdictions. Professional knowledge will increasingly be acquired through digital archives and computer simulations, and professional expertise will increasingly be organized and implemented through the decision trees, search algorithms, and menu structures of "helper" software. The digital revolution may reconfigure the market for professional services, too, as online quality ratings and price comparators computerize and depersonalize the construction of professional reputations, and as telemedicine expands the scope of practice beyond the spatial boundaries of bricks-and-mortar workplaces and flesh-and-blood communities. Even face-to-face workplace relations may change, as skills at the bedside vie with skills at the keyboard, and as dexterity with laboratory rats competes against dexterity with computer mice—a change which has already become evident in certain specialties.[1] The other chapters in this volume shed light on these and other ways in which information technology, qua technology, promises to reshape the understanding of professionalism among medical practitioners.

As great and often wrenching as these transformations may be, however, we must also consider the possibility that IT may exert its greatest impact on medical professionalism not directly, by changing what practitioners do, but indirectly, by changing with whom they collaborate in doing it. As the sociologist Andrew Abbott has famously observed, professional occupations form a "system," in which the fates of different professions (and hence professionalisms) are linked, sometimes competitively, sometimes cooperatively.[2] Nowhere is this more true than in health care, a field where the practitioners of multiple clinical and, increasingly, administrative professions work in close proximity and in tight coordination to provide crucial time-sensitive care. Thus, to understand medical professionalism in the information age, one must look beyond the absorption of IT into medicine itself, to consider how the introduction of IT may restructure the larger "system of professions" that constitutes the health care enterprise as a whole.

As other chapters in this volume illustrate, clinical IT poses a number of significant governance challenges for health care relations, implicating critical issues of integrity, integration, and control.[3] These governance challenges can—and to some extent no doubt will—be resolved by a range of essentially non-professional (or even anti-professional) social structures, such as market competition and bureaucratic oversight. The history and the current direction of American health care, however, suggest that one likely consequence of the rising prominence of health information, health information technology, and health information technology governance will be a concomitant rise in the prominence of new health-information professions. This chapter lays out some preliminary thoughts—and some tentative evidence—on what these new professions will be, who will be their members, and how those members will conceptualize their work, their workplaces, and their own "medical professionalism." We begin by enunciating a sociological account of professionalism, not as an idealistic aspiration but as a distinctive type of occupational structure. We then assess the state of today's health information occupations against this archetype, to determine where and to what degree new health information professions may be emerging. Finally, we consider possible futures for professionalism and professionalization in the health information field, and we briefly speculate on how these futures might shape the impact of information technology on the professionalism of the health care sector's more longstanding and familiar occupational groups.

What Are "Professions" and Why Do They Matter?

To put the emergence of the new health information professions into context, it may be helpful to begin with a few words about the sociology of the professions more generally.[4] Although scholarship on professions is hardly all of one piece, a number of themes are sufficiently prevalent and relevant to merit comment here. In particular, the occupations that we commonly think of as professions generally share a number of core features, and these features generally act to give the professions substantial power as institution-builders—and substantial stability and resilience as institutions in their own right.[5]

Core Features

Early approaches to the sociology of the professions relied heavily on empirical generalization, seeking to abstract a set of defining attributes from scrutiny of the "core" professions—medicine, law, and the ministry.[6] The motivating debates of that era have receded somewhat over time, but the archetype that they left behind remains fairly well accepted today. Actual professions may comport with this template in varying degrees, but over the past half century the basic criteria have become a touchstone for advocates and critics alike. Specifically, most accounts of the professions assume that these occupations share at least the following eight traits:[7]

1. Uncertainty: Professions address vital sources of uncertainty and disorder in social life, such as physical disease (medicine), spiritual salvation (ministry), and social power (law).
2. Knowledge: Professions address these uncertainties by developing and applying coherent bodies of abstract formal knowledge. Although many occupations involve practical judgment and technical skill, professions stand apart in constructing more general conceptual systems, from which practitioners can derive knowledge-based solutions even for unprecedented events.
3. Training: New entrants acquire the profession's body of knowledge through extensive training and socialization in formal educational programs, practical apprenticeships, or both.
4. Autonomy: Professionals value discretion and claim autonomy from lay controls. Lacking the specialized knowledge to determine a proper

course of action, lay clients (and lay administrators) are ill-equipped to question or evaluate professional performance, and must consequently defer to professional prescriptions.

5. Ethics: Despite (or because of) their autonomy from extra-professional oversight, professions cultivate intra-professional restraints—internalized norms, collegial reputations, and formal codes of conduct—that impose ethical duties both toward clients and toward fellow professionals.

6. World view: Professional knowledge and professional ethics often intersect to create a distinctive world view[8]—a predisposition to focus on certain problems, certain solutions, and certain explanations rather than on others. Because professional work often occurs in domains of substantial ambiguity, different world views can lead different professions to approach the same situations in very different ways.

7. Selectivity: Professions seek to control the supply of practitioners and the standards for entry into practice. Typical controls include admissions criteria before training, performance demands during training, and (re)certification requirements after training.

8. Jurisdiction: Professions seek to specify, protect, and extend the range or "jurisdiction" of their practice. In particular, professions often enlist state authority to define certain activities as being solely within the profession's own unique competence, and to exclude unauthorized practitioners, by force of law.

Significantly, despite substantial (albeit tacit) consensus about the elements that set the professions apart from other occupations, the literature on professions has long been split over how and why these traits generally appear in conjunction with one another. Since at least the mid-1970s, two opposing camps have dominated the intellectual landscape. The first view, usually labeled "functionalist," emphasizes professional knowledge, training, and ethics, to paint a relatively favorable image of professionals as highly skilled experts who grapple with crucial technical challenges beyond the ken of most laypersons.[9] In this view, when uncertainty and disorder imperil social survival, professions step to the ramparts: professions develop abstract knowledge to address the threat; professions train and certify practitioners to wield that knowledge; and professions promulgate and embrace ethical codes to ensure that the resulting expertise is used only for the public good.

The second view, usually labeled "critical," emphasizes professional autonomy, selectivity, and jurisdictional control, to paint a much more jaundiced image of professionals as self-serving monopolists who co-opt state authority in parochial projects of market control and group mobility.[10] In this view, uncertainty and disorder are nothing more than convenient pretexts for professional self-aggrandizement: Professions manufacture narratives of social peril and professional competence merely to justify the profession's own political influence and workplace authority; professions create accreditation, admission, and licensure standards merely to symbolize professional expertise and to restrict market supply; and professions disseminate codes of ethics merely to avoid external scrutiny and to restrain internal competition.

Between these stark poles, the literature on the professions offers a wide array of nuances, gray areas, and attempted syntheses. However, the poles continue to matter, at least in part because they reflect an important real-world ambivalence: The functionalist view captures the soaring "professionalism" that each profession's leaders vocally (and often sincerely) extol as a path to service, dignity, and self-fulfillment; the critical view captures the creeping "professionalization" that many laypeople—and many competing professions— vocally (and often sincerely) lament as a path to exploitation, exclusion, and client disempowerment.

Professions as Institution-Builders

Functionalist and conflict theories clearly differ in the relative priority that they accord to particular "core" attributes of professionalism, and in the way that they piece the overall constellation of attributes together into a logically coherent archetype. Nonetheless, most accounts in both traditions agree that the resulting social form—what we know as a profession—possesses a distinctive capacity to maintain internal collegiality (or at least a facade of comity), to generate abstract knowledge-claims, to reap social privileges and material rewards, and to command external trust and authority. These properties position the professions among the most important "institution-builders" of contemporary society.

Since the late 1970s, institutions and institutionalism have moved to the forefront of contemporary scholarship across the social sciences, from sociology[11] to political science[12] to economics[13]—and even into the more "humanistic" disciplines of anthropology and history.[14] Broadly stated, "institutions" are social mechanisms that operate to make behaviors (whether at the individual or the collective level) replicable across time, consistent across sites, predictable across instances, routine across actors, and familiar across audiences.[15] Bureaucratic operating procedures are one obvious example, giving rise to the vernacular usage of "institution" as an appellation for particularly stable, long-lived, and tradition-bound organizations such as museums and universities.

But institutions can also be more informal and micro-interactional (e.g., facing forward in a crowded elevator), or more constitutive and macro-cultural (e.g., the "institution of marriage"). Because institutions facilitate social coordination, they often have a self-enforcing character (e.g., driving on the right-hand side of the road); and because institutions are stable and widely known, they often become the taken-for-granted backdrop of daily life (e.g., the seven-day week). But although institutions may become reified, naturalized, and recalcitrant to change, they remain fundamentally social constructs, generated only by human interaction, reproduced only by human compliance, and forever open to reform by human resistance and entrepreneurship.[16]

W. Richard Scott usefully suggests that institutions can be seen as being supported by three empirically interconnected but conceptually distinct "pillars": a *regulative* pillar composed of explicit, coercive rules and sanctions that play on actors' rational self-interests; a *normative* pillar composed of internalized ethical principles and commitments that play on actors' values and moral beliefs; and a *cognitive* pillar composed of tacit, often taken-for-granted accounts, typologies, and definitions that play on actors' mental models of, and expectations for, social reality.[17] Each of these pillars can serve to buttress and stabilize institutionalized social practices, and each can also provide leverage for "institutional entrepreneurs" to construct, promote, and legitimate new social practices that, with sufficient persistence and popularization, may eventually become institutionalized in their own right.[18] Although the balance among the three may vary from one institution to another, together the regulative, normative, and cognitive pillars represent the key building blocks of durable and resilient (or, more pessimistically, recalcitrant and constraining) social structures.

Within this institutionalist framework, professions stand among the most important institutionalizing agents of the modern world, often with privileged access to each of the three major institutional pillars.[19] Modern societies increasingly seem uncomfortable reposing great powers of social control and social transformation in the hands of "mere" laypeople. Thus, regulative tools are increasingly given over to professional militaries, professional police, and professional judges; normative tools are entrusted to professional clergy, professional ethicists, professional therapists, and professional coaches; cognitive tools, to professional scientists, professional analysts, and professional informaticians. But equally important, almost every profession, regardless of its core jurisdiction, enjoys a privileged right to deploy various regulative, normative, and cognitive devices in the service of its particular, socially authorized mission. Thus, for example, doctors are empowered to fight disease not only through the cognitive/scientific techniques of experimentation, testing, diagnosis, and prognosis, but also through the normative/ethical techniques of counseling, prescription, and "wellness-promotion," and at least occasionally through the regulative/coercive techniques of involuntary commitment, quarantine, and physical or pharmacological restraint.[20]

Not surprisingly, each profession tends to deploy the tools at its disposal in a distinctive way, governed by the profession's unique bundle of material interests, ethical commitments, and mental models—that is, by its "professional world view." As a result, the mix of professions that are active in any given sector of social life becomes an important determinant of how events in that sector will unfold, both at the micro level of daily workplace encounters and at the macro level of long-run historical trends. Indeed, this fact can often be exploited by institutional entrepreneurs who recognize that one way to change the trajectory of a sector is to change the collection of professionals who are authorized to be present when decisions get made.[21] This is a point to which we will return at the close of this chapter.

Professions as Built Institutions

Without detracting from the foregoing depiction of professions as institutionalizing agents, our current exploration of the emerging "health information professions" rests at least as heavily on a second element of the institutionalist picture: professions are not only institutionalizers but also institutions in their own right. Thus, the task of building the profession itself is foremost among the institution-building tasks that most professions face. This task is often termed the "professional project,"[22] and it involves concerted, persistent collective action in pursuit of at least three interrelated goals: identification, legitimation, and enclosure.

First, champions of professionalization must generate a sense of commonality, solidarity, and collective identity among practitioners. At times, this *identification* can emerge organically out of shared experiences, including shared frictions with other professions in the workplace.[23] But more often a sense of commonality requires active nurturing that involves all three institutional pillars: Work practices need to be standardized to give rise to common experiences and common values; job titles, technical language, and norms of dress and address need to be promulgated to give rise to common cognitive schemas and common social identities; and career ladders, client relations, funding streams, and patterns of authority and deference need to be regularized to give rise to common incentives and common interests. Researchers often overlook the importance of these tasks, because the process of identity formation usually begins well before anyone in the outside world notices the existence of an occupation to be professionalized. But the building of a shared social identity is nonetheless crucial—precisely because, in its absence, there will be no collectivity to take the collective actions that further professionalization demands.[24]

Once a sense of identification has begun to emerge (but often before a professional identity is fully developed), the nascent profession must *legitimate* itself to external audiences.[25] Again, all three pillars may be involved.[26] Legitimation is, in part, a matter of forming stable exchange relations with powerful patrons. Nascent professions frequently need to make a case that they can bring in business, enhance efficiency, open markets, satisfy customers, reduce workloads, control legal risks, garner grants, and, in general, pay their way. But legitimation is not purely a matter of creating a positive return on investment for the powers that be. Legitimation almost always rests on judgments of normative propriety and cognitive comprehensibility, as well. Thus, would-be professions generally seek to construct and popularize cultural accounts that: (a) "naturalize" the new profession's domain, routines, and internal organization;[27] (b) identify a social "need" that the profession addresses; (c) explicate the unique knowledge-base and ethical commitments that make the profession a particularly trustworthy, competent, and suitable vehicle for addressing that need; and (d) articulate a social problem or crisis, either actual or incipient, that demands that the profession be further authorized and empowered.[28]

Finally, to persist and to hold its own within the larger system of the professions, an occupation must *enclose* its core jurisdiction.[29] It must, in Richard Abel's phrase, establish control over both "production *by* professionals" (i.e., the scope, nature, and terms of practice) and "production *of* professionals" (i.e., the criteria for recruitment, training, and admission to practice).[30] While the enclosure of professional domains is often caricatured as being primarily a matter of establishing monopolistic market control,[31] it (like the other aspects of the professional project) is in fact a more multifaceted institution-building enterprise, with the nascent profession seeking to secure and institutionalize not only a claim to material resources but also a set of parallel claims to social deference and cultural authority. Much of the process is, as the market-control metaphor suggests, regulative: new professions frequently enlist the state or other powerful entities—insurance companies, banks, universities, charitable foundations, and the like—in creating demand or in restricting supply. The archetype is formal licensure, in which a state regulator (a) limits practice to licensed professionals; (b) authorizes an accreditation system to certify licensees; and (c) requires that certain mandated activities be conducted with the assistance of licensed staff. However, more modest arrangements are also quite common. For example, powerful entities can often (sometimes inadvertently) promote the growth of a profession simply by creating a sense of threat or uncertainty around a topic that happens to lie within that profession's professed competence. Several scholars have noted this dynamic with regard to the impact of employment law on the growth of the "personnel professions"— human resource managers, labor lawyers, career counselors, and so on.[32] And, as described below, a similar process may be at work in the impact of health privacy law on the growth of the health information professions.

The effectiveness of such non-mandatory interventions highlights the fact that professions often pursue enclosure through normative and cognitive, as well as regulative, channels. Normatively, professions claim a place at the table as representatives of important cultural ideals, such as efficiency and innovation (e.g., management consultants), legality and formalization (e.g., lawyers), health and safety (e.g., physicians), or information and control (e.g., accountants). Cognitively, professions secure their position by becoming incorporated into the taken-for-granted constitutive scripts and schemas for various types of action: In finance, "due diligence" implies a review of legal documents, and a review of legal documents implies the retention of a lawyer; in health information, one could imagine that "quality control" might imply a statistical summary of patient outcomes, and a statistical summary of patient outcomes might imply the retention of a statistician.

Although one can analytically decompose professional projects into identification, legitimation, and enclosure, one must also recognize that these phenomena often occur together, at the same time, and in the same empirical loci. Moreover, in most cases, the institutionalization of new professions, like institutional change in general, proceeds through a creative leveraging of preexisting institutional structures, and each preexisting institution may bear on multiple facets of the professional project. Early leaders create professional associations to promote identification, enhance legitimacy, and pursue enclosure—all within an established organizational form (the nonprofit membership association) recognized by law and popularized by previous generations of trade associations in the organizational environment.[33] Similarly, professional training programs simultaneously develop alumni networks (identification), canonize systems of knowledge and ethics (legitimation), and implement selection, certification, and accreditation criteria (enclosure)—all in close collaboration with established educational institutions such as universities and standardized testing services. Both legitimation and enclosure often proceed in tandem with the social control agendas of established state agencies; and naturalization, taken-for-grantedness and (perceived) efficacy all emerge primarily through routinized interactions within established workplaces within established firms.

Thus, although the long-term impact of a new profession can be substantial, the early stages of most professional projects go almost unnoticed, except perhaps by their most zealous advocates. Rather than appearing ex nihilo as an invading horde on the horizon, most new professions gradually coalesce in the interstices of existing social structures,[34] occasionally nudging and jostling other professions for jurisdictional elbow room,[35] but rarely fighting grand pitched battles, until the war is already effectively won. For this reason, emerging professions are often overlooked or underestimated, even though the signs of their growth are merely hidden in plain sight.

This, we would argue, is precisely the condition of the health information field today. In the pages that follow, we explore the signs of emerging health-information professionalism, and we speculate on the implications of this development for the complex system of professions that makes up the modern health care sector.

Meet the HIPsters

What empirical evidence might bear on these theoretical suppositions? A full investigation would necessarily go well beyond the limits of the present chapter. However, even a casual perusal of various publicly available records suggests that the health information field is becoming increasingly professionalized, and that inter-professional dynamics in the field are becoming increasingly rich, complex, and consequential. Health information workers are reconceptualizing themselves as health information *professionals* (HIPs), and whether tacitly or explicitly, these HIPs and the proto-professions that they compose are striving to carve out viable niches alongside the more established professions in the health care landscape. Here, we present a smorgasbord of empirical evidence that suggests the basic contours of this shifting terrain.

Emergence and Identification

As a starting point, evidence of the growth of the health-information *workforce* abounds: According to the U.S. Bureau of Labor Statistics (BLS),[36] the decade from 1997 to 2006 saw a rapid rise in the number of jobs in the health care sector both for computer specialists (up 49 percent) and for medical records and health information technicians (up 77 percent).[37] These growth rates far outpace growth in the sector as a whole, in health care administration as a whole, and in the core clinical professions. Moreover, even in the absence of major new public policy initiatives, job growth among health care-sector computer specialists is expected to continue to equal or exceed job growth among both clinicians and non-IT administrators throughout the coming decade, with an additional 16,500 jobs being added by 2016.

Significantly, table 8.1 also shows some evidence of professional upgrading: The number of low-end health information jobs (filing clerks, data-entry workers, etc.) is declining precipitously, even while the number of high-end jobs (information systems administrators, analysts, and programmers) rises. And although job growth in the middle tier—the category that the BLS labels "medical records and health information technicians"—significantly outpaced the other two segments from 1997 to 2006, it is expected to lag behind the rapidly growing high-end segment from 2006 to 2016. Apparently, employment in the health information field is not only growing, but it is growing most rapidly in the upper echelons.

HIP worksites

The BLS data also shed some light on the contours of the health information workplace. Figure 8.1 depicts the relative distribution of low-end, technician-level, and high-end HIPs across ambulatory, hospital, and long-term care settings. At least two patterns are noteworthy: The first is the concentration of low-end HIPs in ambulatory care (62 percent of the low-end total), and the concentration of high-end HIPs in hospitals (76 percent of the high-end total); the second is the overall low number of HIPs of any kind in long-term care settings (only 7 percent of the overall total), and the almost exclusive preponderance of technician-level workers among the few HIPs who are present (86 percent of the long-term care total).

Figure 8.2 depicts average annual salaries across these same skill levels and worksites. The patterns here are less dramatic. As might be expected, high-end HIPs consistently earn more than twice as much as low-end HIPs ($60,000–$70,000 versus $20,000–$25,000). Somewhat more surprisingly, the earnings of tech-level HIPs ($25,000–$30,000) are much closer to low-end HIPs than to high, an indication that the BLS's "health information technicians" category may be a relatively poor proxy for the HIP workforce as a whole. Also somewhat surprisingly, HIP incomes vary only slightly by work setting: Hospitals are the most lucrative setting for all three groups, by a small margin; for low-end and tech-level workers, long-term care comes next, and ambulatory care last; while for high-end workers, ambulatory care comes next and long-term care last. Significantly, however, these differences across worksites are dwarfed by the differences across occupational groups, suggesting that work tasks rather than work settings are currently the primary drivers of inequality within the field.[38]

Table 8.1   Historical and Projected Health Care Sector[a] Employment in Selected Occupations, 1997–2016

Occupation	2006 Mean Annual Income	1997 Number	2006 Number	2016 Number (projected)	1997–2006 Percent Change	2006–2016 Percent Change
Computer specialists	$57,487	47,460	70,698	87,132	48.96	23.25
Managers and administrators[b]	$73,080	(13,621)	20,347	24,977	49.38	22.76
Analysts, programmers and software engineers[c]	$64,832	25,780	35,412	44,712	37.36	26.26
Medical records and health information technicians	$29,222	80,590	142,428	168,900	76.73	18.59
Filing, data-entry, etc.[d]	$23,387	164,720	112,991	82,578	−31.40	−26.92
All management and administrative occupations	$81,204	476,610	412,674	481,577	−13.41	16.70
All diagnosing and treating practitioners[e]	$78,514	2,730,310	3,269,011	4,023,559	19.73	23.08
Physicians and surgeons	$160,219	407,170	467,633	547,518	14.85	17.08
Registered nurses	$59,763	1,719,710	2,072,391	2,594,522	20.51	25.19
Total health care employment, all occupations	$43,376	10,744,760	13,621,400	16,575,600	26.77	21.69

[a]1997 2-digit SIC industry 8000; 2006 3-digit NAICS industries 621, 622, 623

[b]2006 OES codes 11-3021, 15-1061, 15-1071

[c]1997 OES codes 25102, 25105, 25108; 2006 OES codes 15-1030, 15-1051, 15-1021, 15-1081

[d]1997 OES codes 55321, 56017, 56000, 56011; 2006 OES codes 43-4071, 439021, 43-9020, 43-9011

[e]1997 OES codes 32102, 32105, 32108, 32111, 32113, 32199, 32302, 32305, 32308, 32311. 32314, 32317, 32399, 32502, 32511, 32517, 32521,

Source: Data on which table is based obtained from www.bls.gov/oes/.

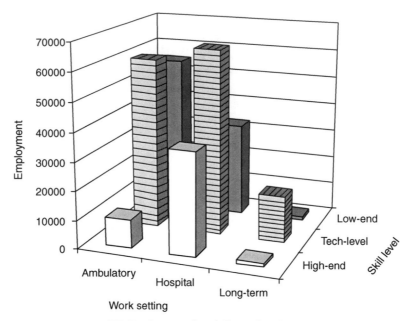

Figure 8.1   HIP Employment by Skill Level and Work Setting, 2006
Source: Data on which figure is based obtained from www.bls.gov/oes/.

HIP associations

High market demand and a growing body of practitioners may facilitate the emergence of a professional project, but raw numbers alone are rarely enough to bring such a project to fruition. Professional projects are social movements of a sort[39] requiring mutual awareness and collective action in order to succeed. One key marker—and motor—of such mobilization is the formation of new professional and trade associations.[40] On this index, as on simple employment, the health information field displays striking activity: In the past twenty-five years, a veritable alphabet soup of such associations has emerged, all catering to the health information management (HIM) workforce in one way or another. An unsystematic search of Web sites and press releases uncovers at least half a dozen independent professional bodies, and another half-dozen special-interest subunits of other longstanding professional associations, such as the American Academy of Family Physicians' Center for Health Information Technology (CHIT) and the American Society for Information Science and Technology's Special Interest Group on Medical Informatics (SIGMED). These professional bodies often work closely with a dozen or so industry groups representing various segments of the emerging health information technology marketplace, and

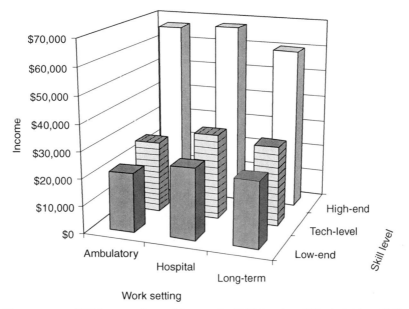

Figure 8.2   HIP Average Annual Income by Skill Level and Work Setting, 2006
Source: Data on which figure is based obtained from www.bls.gov/oes/.

with a similar number of groups focusing on the issues of health privacy and computer security.

By most accounts, the most prominent of the HIP associations are the American Health Information Management Association (AHIMA), the Healthcare Information and Management Systems Society (HIMSS), the American Medical Informatics Association (AMIA), the College of Healthcare Information Management Executives (CHIME), the Association of Medical Directors of Information Systems (AMDIS), and the American Academy of Professional Coders (AAPC). The first three (AHIMA, HIMSS, and AMIA) have pursued generalist strategies,[41] while the others have focused more narrowly on particular segments of the emerging field. Table 8.2 and figure 8.3 present a capsule summary and timeline of these entities and their histories.

Of the six, AHIMA is by far the oldest, having been created by the American College of Surgeons in 1928 (under the name "Association of Record Librarians of North America") to "elevate the standards of clinical records in hospitals and other medical institutions."[42] The organization passed through several name changes in its history, becoming the American Association of Medical Record Librarians in 1938 and the American Medical Record Association in 1970. As the association's Web site notes, the succession of names reflects

Table 8.2 Summary of Selected Health Information Professional and Trade Organizations

Organization name	Founding date	Current size	History	Core constituency
AHIMA-American Health Information Management Association	1991	51,000	Founded as Assoc. of Record Librarians of N.Am. (ARLNA), 1928; renamed Am. Assoc. of Med. Record Librarians (AAMRL), 1938; renamed Am. Med. Record Assoc. (AMRA), 1970; renamed AHIMA, 1991.	Medical records professionals
HIMSS - Healthcare Information and Management Systems Society	1986	20,000	Founded as Hospital Mgmt. Systems Soc'y (HMSS), 1961; affiliates with AHA, 1966; renamed HIMSS, 1986; becomes independent of AHA, 1989; absorbs CHIM 2002; absorbs CPRI-HOST, 2003; absorbs AFEHCT, 2006.	IT professionals and industry partners
AMIA - American Medical Informatics Association	1990	3,000	Formed by 1990 merger of: Symposium on Computer Applications in Medical Care (SCAMC), founded 1977 Am. College of Med. Informatics (ACMI), founded 1984 Am. Assoc. for Med. Systems and Informatics (AAMSI), formed by 1981 merger of: Soc'y for Computer Med. (SCM), founded 1972 Soc'y for Adv. Med. Systems (SAMS), founded 1975.	Informatics researchers
CHIME - College of Healthcare Information Management Executives	1992	1,254	Initially sponsored by HIMSS and CHIM	CIOs
AMDIS - Association of Medical Directors of Information Systems	1997	1,980		CMIO physicians

Organization	Year	Members	Notes	Role
AAPC - American Academy of Professional Coders	1988	74,000		Coders
CHIM - Center for Healthcare Information Management	1986		Founded within AHA in 1986; became independent in 1989; merged into HIMSS in 2002	Funding channel
CPRI - Computer-based Patient Record Institute	1992		Merged with HOST to form CPRI-HOST in 2000; absorbed into HIMSS in 2003	Industry advocacy
HOST - Healthcare Open Systems and Trials	1994		Merged with CPRI to form CPRI-HOST in 2000; absorbed into HIMSS in 2003	Benchmarking
JHITA - Joint Healthcare Information Technology Alliance	1997		Founded as joint venture of HIMSS, CHIME and CHIM; joined by AHIMA and AMIA in 1998	Clearinghouse/advocacy
AFEHCT - Association for Electronic Health Care Transactions	1992		Absorbed by HIMSS in 2006	Vendor advocacy

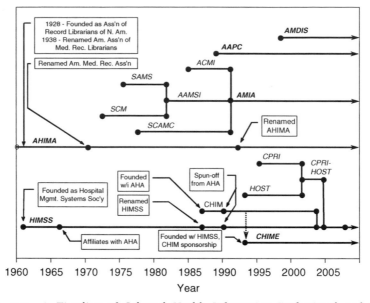

Figure 8.3   A Timeline of Selected Health Information Professional and Trade Organizations

"the evolution of the profession"—from an offshoot of librarianship, to the handling of patient clinical records, to the management of health information in any form, in any setting, and at any stage in the continuum of care.[43] Today, AHIMA boasts over 50,000 members, working in a wide array of roles.[44] Most significantly, with the advent of the Health Insurance Portability and Accountability Act (HIPAA), AHIMA has become an important forum for privacy officers, as well as for more traditional health information administrators. The organization offers a wide array of professional certifications in health information management, medical coding, health privacy and security, and health data analysis.[45] Yet, despite its increasingly broad portfolio, AHIMA continues to have a core constituency of medical records administrators, and as a result, it tends to reflect the data-focused orientation of "information management" (IM) somewhat more than either the hardware orientation of "information technology" (IT), the clinical orientation of medicine, or the enterprise-administration orientation of "management information systems" (MIS).

The second oldest of the leading HIP associations is the Healthcare Information and Management Systems Society (HIMSS).[46] Founded in 1961 as the Hospital Management Systems Society, HIMSS spent twenty-three years of its history (1966–1989) as an affiliated subunit of the American Hospital Association (AHA).[47] Both its original name (which was changed to HIMSS in

1986) and its long affiliation with the AHA signal an affinity with the concerns of MIS administrators in hospitals and other large health care organizations. Its early leaders also shared a commitment to applying industrial engineering principles to the health care workplace (a movement known at the time as "hospital management engineering"), giving the organization a stronger technology focus than some of its counterparts.[48] With a current membership of approximately 20,000, HIMSS is less than half the size of AHIMA; however, like AHIMA, HIMSS offers a professional credential (the Certified Professional in Healthcare Information and Management Systems or CPHIMS) and provides various professional development opportunities for its individual members.[49] HIMSS has also broadened its outreach in recent years, particularly in the two decades since its separation from the AHA. In particular, HIMSS has been noticeably more aggressive than AHIMA in building links to industry (including IT vendors as well as health care providers), in developing an explicit policy-advocacy capacity, and in pursuing mergers with other professional and trade associations in the field.[50] In 2002, for example, HIMSS absorbed the Center for Healthcare Information Management (CHIM), a fellow AHA spin-off that had originally been formed to facilitate the involvement of vendors and consultants in the AHA's health information technology advocacy efforts; in 2003, HIMSS absorbed CPRI-HOST (Computer-based Patient Record Institute— Healthcare Open Systems and Trials), an industry group combining advocacy for computerized patient records with implementation benchmarking and demonstration projects; and in 2006, HIMSS absorbed the Association for Electronic Health Care Transactions (AFEHCT), a vendor-based advocacy group pursuing public policies conducive to electronic data interchange (EDI). This blending of industry advocacy and professional development arguably makes HIMSS the most generalized of the major players in the field, although it also somewhat dilutes the organization's identity as a profession-builder.

The final generalist HIP entity is the American Medical Informatics Association (AMIA).[51] Founded in 1990, AMIA melded three earlier health informatics associations: the Symposium on Computer Applications in Medical Care (SCAMC, founded in 1977), the American Association for Medical Systems and Informatics (AAMSI, founded in 1981),[52] and the American College of Medical Informatics (ACMI, founded in 1984).[53] Perhaps more strongly than AHIMA and HIMSS, AMIA's roots lie in academia, and it continues to emphasize "thought leadership" over skill certification or lobbying.[54] This orientation can be seen in the relatively high proportion of academics among AMIA's officers,[55] as well as in the operation within AMIA of an Academic Strategic Leadership Council and an Academic Forum "to provide guidance, support, and advocacy for academic programs in . . . health informatics."[56] With slightly under 4,000 members, AMIA is much smaller than either AHIMA or HIMSS. Nonetheless, as the rise of health information work has increased the demand for medical informaticians in government and industry settings, AMIA has paralleled its larger counterparts in expanding its mission and diversifying its membership. Today, less than 30 percent of AMIA's members work in academic settings,[57] and according to an AMIA spokesperson, less than half hold M.D. or Ph.D. degrees, with the rest being "all across the board." AMIA has also become an active advocate for the professional status of medical informatics practitioners, winning acceptance into the Council of Medical Specialty Societies (CMSS) in November 2006.

The remaining three core HIP associations, the College of Healthcare Information Management Executives (CHIME), the Association of Medical Directors of Information Systems (AMDIS), and the American Academy of Professional Coders (AAPC) are both newer and more specialized than AHIMA, HIMSS, and AMIA. Consistent with the common organizational phenomenon of "resource partitioning,"[58] as the field's generalist associations have consolidated, interstitial niches have opened for more focused entities that cater to the distinctive needs of particular constituencies. Of the three, CHIME is arguably the most closely aligned with the sector's power structure, having been founded in 1992 with direct HIMSS and CHIM support and with the active involvement of several prominent HIMSS and CHIM leaders.[59] CHIME's membership is explicitly restricted to chief information officers and others "in charge of IS for major divisions and/or regions of large corporate or integrated delivery systems, . . . insurance organizations, and other healthcare-related organizations."[60] This restriction makes CHIME a small but influential player, and the 1,200-member organization frequently leverages its influence through collaboration with its larger, more generalist counterparts. Thus in 1997, for example, CHIME joined HIMSS and CHIM in founding the Joint Healthcare Information Technology Alliance (JHITA), to coordinate legislative/regulatory advocacy and industry education. By the next year, AHIMA and AMIA had joined as well, creating an important vehicle for coordinating collective action during the HIPAA rulemaking period.[61]

The final two associations, AMDIS and AAPC, represent health information professionals in more tenuous positions. With close to 2,000 individual members, AMDIS, like CHIME, serves a relatively small slice of the professional field.[62] In contrast to CHIME, however, AMDIS's core constituency is the chief medical information officer (CMIO), essentially a liaison role between the information systems function (represented by the chief information officer, CIO) and the clinical function (represented by the chief medical officer, CMO) in large health care organizations. CMIOs are often practicing physicians who have chosen to become "IT champions," and their primary identity is generally as clinicians.[63] Yet they can find themselves in an awkward political position if the medical and administrative sides of their organizations disagree over the purpose or value of clinical IT. Mediating this jurisdictional tension represents an important component of AMDIS's agenda.

AAPC's position in the HIP professional project is, if anything, even more fraught. With close to 75,000 members,[64] AAPC is ironically both the largest and also the most marginal of the core HIP bodies. The "professional coders" whom it represents are a relatively weak occupational group, specializing in the "back office" task of assigning standardized codes to clinical diagnoses and treatments, in order to facilitate claims processing. Although their work is painstaking and crucial to the functioning of the health insurance system, in most work settings they have moderate incomes, little supervisory authority, and only limited opportunities for advancement.[65] It is perhaps noteworthy that AAPC is the one HIP association whose core constituency might *suffer* economically if the HIP field's favored policy agenda—universal implementation of standardized electronic health record systems, with computer provider order-entry and electronic data interchange capabilities—were to come to fruition. It is also perhaps noteworthy that AAPC is the only major HIP association whose Web site prominently features a "Member Bill of Rights."

These differences notwithstanding, perhaps the most noteworthy feature of the HIP landscape is the virtual absence of overt conflict—or even commensalistic competition—among the leading associations. The one exception is in the market for "certified coder" credentials, where AHIMA and AAPC are both active; but even here, some tacit coordination exists, with AHIMA focusing on hospital-based coding, while AAPC focuses on coders working in physician practices.[66] More generally, the core HIP associations share similar policy agendas and they routinely collaborate on a wide range of advocacy, professionalization, and market-expansion projects. Many individuals belong to (and hold leadership roles in) more than one association, and the speaker and exhibitor lists for their conventions overlap substantially. The widespread perception seems to be that the field as a whole is on the ascendant, and that everyone's energies are best invested in expanding rather than in dividing the pie. Organizational sociology argues that the participants in an emerging industry generally gain more from the additional legitimation that each new entrant

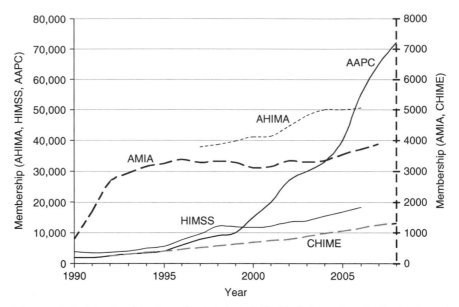

Figure 8.4   Membership Growth of Selected Health Information Professional and Trade Organizations

provides than they lose from the additional competition that each new entrant creates.[67] For the moment, at least, this clearly seems to be the case among the core HIP associations. Figure 8.4 displays the growth trajectories of several of these bodies, for those years where data is available. The trends in all cases are unambiguously upward, although the precise timing of spurts and lulls differs.[68]

Expertise and Legitimation

Numerical prevalence, collective self-awareness, and organizational mobilization are important initial hurdles for a professional project; however, an additional crucial step involves the construction and enactment of a legitimating rationale to explain the profession's activities and to justify the profession's privileges. Most effective professional rationales seek, in one way or another, to integrate narratives of complex abstract knowledge, pressing social need, and altruistic practitioner ethics. The work of building such an account has been under way in the HIP field for quite some time; and whether tacitly or explicitly, this legitimation task occupies a high position on the agendas of virtually all the field's major professional associations. Although the legitimation process is far less advanced than in health care's long-dominant clinical and administrative professions, it has certainly advanced far enough to be readily palpable to HIP practitioners and readily visible to outside observers.

Conferences and conventions

Perhaps the simplest marker of legitimation activity in the HIP field is the proliferation of professional conferences and conventions. As sites for social networking, conferences could easily be caricatured as simply an additional element of the self-identification process described above. Conferences, however, can also serve as essential venues for several key legitimation activities. Most obviously, conferences disseminate new knowledge, foster intra-professional dialogue, and provide a forum for aspirational and inspirational rhetoric, all crucial components of building a shared sense of professional expertise, purpose, and social responsibility. Conferences also offer a test of the profession's broader social relevance, through their ability to attract outside sponsors and exhibitors. Finally, conferences (especially recurring annual conferences) help to bolster the profession's aura of permanence and taken-for-grantedness. Thus, conferences represent a useful indicator of several aspects of professional legitimation.

By this metric, the HIP field is doing well. All six of the major HIP associations hold one or more annually scheduled conventions (AMIA and AAPC hold three and CHIME holds two), as does the Agency for Healthcare Research and Quality, the federal government's leading clearinghouse and funder for clinical IT research.[69] Interspersed among these twelve recurring events are numerous occasional mini-conferences, and an even larger number of "audio conferences," "podcasts," and "webinars." An unsystematic search of HIP-related Web sites finds at least eight such mini-conferences and at least twenty-eight such virtual events in the first six months of 2009 alone. Although historical data on the number of attendees and exhibitors at these various convocations is hard to come by, CHIME provides attendance numbers for the full history of its spring and fall CIO Forums,[70] and HIMSS provides both attendance and exhibitor figures for its annual convention going back to the late 1980s.[71] These trajectories, plotted in figure 8.5, show strong growth for both gatherings—although, interestingly, HIMSS's attendance appears to have leveled off temporarily during the Y2K/HIPAA implementation period, perhaps due to the flurry of competing events at the time.

Journals

A second important marker of a new profession's developing knowledge base is the proliferation of scholarly journals and other publications. By this metric, again, the HIP field appears to be well along in its legitimation project. The three major generalist HIP associations (AHIMA, HIMSS, and AMIA) each publish regular peer-reviewed journals, as well as numerous white papers, books,

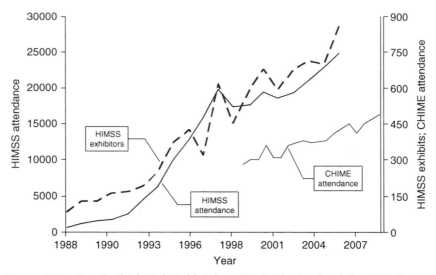

Figure 8.5   Growth of Selected Health Information Professional and Trade Conferences

manuals, and surveys. But this only scratches the surface of the available literature. A more extensive search finds at least thirty-eight HIP-related serials that are currently active, and at least twelve more that have gone out of print.[72] Figure 8.6 plots the total number of journals in print, as well as the number of foundings, failures, and name changes from 1945 to the present. After a slow start in the 1960s, the count of active journals displays the familiar sigmoid growth pattern that is characteristic of many new organizational populations.[73] Interestingly, though, the count of foundings suggests that new journals were formed primarily during three distinct waves, the first in the mid-1970s, the second in the mid-1980s, and then the third (and largest) in the mid-1990s. The last of these waves seems to have somewhat exceeded the field's carrying capacity: the foundings of the mid-1990s gave way to a burst of failures (and renamings of journals to attract new readers) at the turn of the twenty-first century, with the total number of journals falling back slightly from its 1997–1998 peak.

Significantly, although both the mid-1990s growth spurt and the turn-of-the-century plateau in HIP journal numbers closely parallel the trajectory of HIP association memberships and HIP conference attendance, the longer timespan of the journal data reveals the degree to which the field's cognitive foundations were already being laid in the 1970s and 1980s. Without a more extensive analysis of article contents, it is impossible to determine the degree of intellectual continuity between the three waves of journal-founding activity. Impressionistically, however, the first wave of journals seems to have focused heavily on hardware topics like "computing" and "engineering"; the second

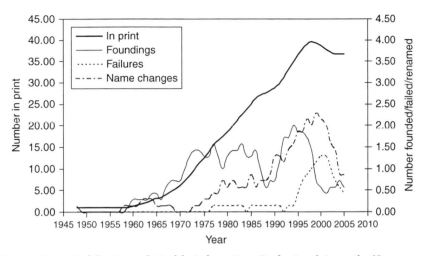

Figure 8.6 Proliferation of Health Information Professional Journals (Seven-year moving averages)

wave, on clinical knowledge-processing topics like "data," "decision-making," and "informatics"; and the third wave on hospital administration and market outreach topics like "information management," "e-health," and "telemedicine." The renamings of journals at the turn of the twenty-first century may also reveal some signs of the field's accelerating quest for professional legitimacy, with several publications adding the more academic-sounding designation "journal" to their titles: Thus, for example, in 1997 *Health Informatics* became the *Health Informatics Journal*; in 2001 *Health Information Management* became the *HIM Journal*; and in 2003 *Health Care on the Internet* became the *Journal of Consumer Health on the Internet*.

Training

Although the proliferation of journals suggests the emergence of a substantial body of abstract knowledge within the HIP field, it says less about the field's capacity to reproduce a self-sustaining corps of professionalized researchers and practitioners to deploy that knowledge. Thus, a third important indicator of professional expertise and legitimation must be the institutionalization of formal training programs within the HIP domain. Several of the leading HIP associations maintain directories of such programs in their focal areas,[74] and judging by numbers alone, this aspect of the HIP project is easily on pace with the aspects discussed above: AHIMA lists twenty-four "approved" training programs in medical coding;[75] AMIA lists eighty-two academic programs in medical informatics;[76] and HIMSS lists forty programs in "HIMSS-related" disciplines.[77]

In addition, in 2004 AHIMA established an independent "Commission on Accreditation for Health Informatics and Information Management Education" (CAHIIM), to provide official accreditation to educational programs in the field. CAHIIM currently lists close to 250 accredited programs at both the associate-degree and baccalaureate level.[78] Combining and reconciling these various lists, one can arrive at a ballpark estimate of approximately 360 HIP training and degree programs, of one sort or another, offering approximately 535 different educational opportunities, at approximately 335 educational institutions nationwide.[79] To put this figure in context, the Liaison Committee on Medical Education (LCME) currently accredits 129 U.S. medical schools,[80] while the National League for Nursing Accrediting Commission (NLNAC) and the Commission on Collegiate Nursing Education (CCNE) together accredit close to 2,000 programs in nursing.[81]

The HIP training picture becomes somewhat less rosy, however, when one looks behind the numbers, to the mix of programs that the various lists comprise. While the sheer prevalence of programs attests to the fact that HIP work is widely perceived as requiring specialized knowledge, the nature of the programs suggests that the magnitude of the requisite knowledge is not always large. Almost two-thirds (65 percent) of the listed programs offer pre-baccalaureate certificates or associate degrees, generally from technical, community, and junior colleges, while only a quarter (26 percent) offer training at the graduate level or above. Moreover, as figure 8.7 demonstrates, the distribution of programs is strikingly bi-modal: The largest block (208 programs) offer only pre-baccalaureate training, while the second largest block (72 programs) offers only post-baccalaureate training. This pattern mirrors the bifurcation described above, between a "low-end" of HIP jobs held by medical coders and health information technicians, and a "high-end" held by medical informaticians and health information administrators. Despite the efforts of some field-level entities (particularly CAHIIM) to span this divide, the evidence from actual training programs suggests that the HIP "body of knowledge" is not currently all of a single piece. Further evidence of this disjointedness comes from the fact that 315 of the 360 listed HIP training programs appear on only one of the four major lists, and a mere six programs appear on three lists or more. It may also be noteworthy that twenty of the 335 educational institutions represented on the combined list provide HIP training not through a single, integrated department or school, but through multiple, independent programs across campus. This pattern reinforces the sense that although HIP expertise is both real and urgently relevant to the contemporary health care system, such expertise has yet to become firmly consolidated into a coherent and discrete body of professional knowledge.

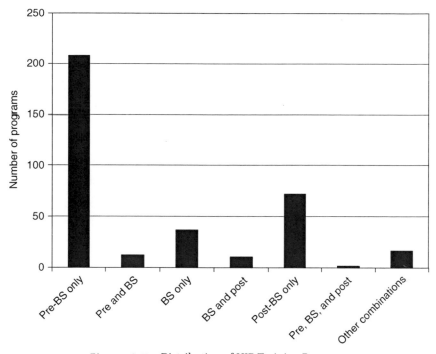

Figure 8.7 Distribution of HIP Training Programs

Ethics

A final crucial factor in the legitimation of a new profession is the formulation, promulgation, and inculcation of a distinctive ethical vision. Professional ethics matter for many normative and policy reasons, of course. However, for the purpose of evaluating the progress of a professional project, the question is less whether practitioners actually *become* more ethical, than whether practitioners and clients alike come to see practice as being ethically freighted. Rhetorically, ethics and expertise are two sides of the same coin: An account of expertise can explain why particular technical services are socially desirable, but an account of expertise alone cannot easily explain why professional practice should be regulated primarily by the profession itself.[82] Thus, to claim control over production by producers, a profession must move from asserting distinctive technical knowledge to asserting distinctive wisdom and judgment— and then on to asserting a distinctive sense of responsibility and a distinctive commitment to altruistic self-control. The classic professional narrative may begin with "only we know how to do this"; but it usually ends with "and only we truly appreciate its gravity—and therefore only we can be trusted to do it responsibly."

The health information professions clearly have not yet developed the elaborate ethical apparatus of more established professions such as medicine, nursing, and law. Discussions of HIP ethics often note the inconsistency and sketchiness of current conceptualizations and the scarcity of concrete mechanisms for self-policing and discipline.[83] Nonetheless, on this dimension as on the dimension of expertise, the HIP professional project appears to be proceeding briskly.

With a few exceptions,[84] academic writings on the distinctive ethical challenges of health information date back no further than the late 1980s.[85] However, the discourse blossomed at the turn of the twenty-first century. In 1997, the American Association for the Advancement of Science (AAAS) produced a path-breaking anthology on *Health Care and Information Ethics*;[86] in 2001, AHIMA sponsored an anthology on *Ethical Challenges in the Management of Health Information*;[87] and between 1998 and 2003, a flurry of essays by Eike-Henner Kluge accompanied the development of the International Medical Informatics Association's (IMIA) 2002 Code of Ethics.[88] The pace of scholarly publication has continued to accelerate in recent years, leaving little doubt that health information poses significant ethical challenges worthy of sustained philosophical inquiry (though there are dissenting views).[89]

However, as AHIMA's and IMIA's early involvement suggests, health information ethics have not been the purview of academics alone. AHIMA and IMIA have both promulgated elaborate ethical codes, the preambles of which offer extensive, theoretically grounded disquisitions on the moral dimensions of health information professionalism.[90] Most of the other major HIP associations have also at least paid lip service to an ethics agenda: AMIA has adopted a substantial IMIA-inspired code of its own and has formed an ongoing working group on "Ethical, Legal, and Social Issues" (ELSI-WG);[91] HIMSS, too, has adopted a lengthy code,[92] albeit one that focuses primarily on members' duties to HIMSS itself, rather than on professional obligations to patients, employers, or the public; and AAPC has adopted a much briefer "Medical Coding Code of Ethics"[93] (see table 8.3).

Of these codes, the AHIMA and IMIA documents offer the clearest sense of a defining HIP vision. In their preambles, both seek to distinguish the ethical situation of HIPs from that of information professionals outside the health care arena. IMIA locates this distinctiveness in the intersecting duties created by, on the one hand, the unique nature of medical records (confidential, yet critical not only to patient care but also to clinical coordination and public health) and, on the other, the unique "web of relationships" in the health care sector (the sometimes conflicting demands from patients, medical practitioners, employer

Table 8.3 **Summary of Selected HIP Ethics Codes**

	AHIMA	IMIA	AMIA	HIMSS	AAPC
Target audience	All HIM professionals	Medical informatics	Medical informatics	HIMSS members	AAPC members
Preamble (word count)	1194	1193	245	148	0
Body (word count)	1985	2412	990	1620	251
General duties					
Competence	✓	✓	✓		✓
Honesty/disclosure	✓	✓	✓	✓	✓
Accountability		✓	✓		
Adherence to law	✓		✓	✓	✓
Continuing education	✓	✓	✓	✓	✓
Advancement of knowledge	✓	✓	✓		
Duties to information					
Security/integrity	✓	✓	✓		
Accuracy	✓	✓			
Timeliness		✓	✓		
Duties to patients					
Dignity/respect for rights	✓	✓	✓		✓
Confidentiality	✓	✓	✓		
Self-determination/ consent	✓	✓			
Notice of data uses, rights		✓	✓		
Duties to co-workers					
Communication	✓	✓	✓		
Teamwork/ responsibility	✓	✓	✓		
Duties to employer					
Honesty	✓	✓	✓	✓	
Loyalty/cooperation		✓	✓		
Proprietary information		✓	✓	✓	
Promote/enforce ethics	✓	✓	✓		✓
Duties to profession					
Enhance status of prof'n	✓	✓	✓	✓	✓
Uphold HIP org's mission	✓			✓	✓
Mentor colleagues	✓	✓			
Duties to society					
Scientific honesty	✓		✓		
Human rights/public health	✓	✓			

(Continued)

Table 8.3   **Continued**

	AHIMA	IMIA	AMIA	HIMSS	AAPC
Service/pro-bono/ education	✓	✓			
Advocate for privacy	✓				
Enforcement provisions					
Enforcement word count	132	0	71	883	26
Disciplinary procedures				✓	
Explicitly non-coercive (in whole or in part)	✓		✓		

organizations, professional bodies, state regulators, and public health agencies).[94] As the AHIMA preamble puts it:

> [M]edical records contain many sacred stories—stories that must be protected on behalf of the individual and the aggregate community of persons served in the healthcare system. . . . Issues include what information should be collected; how the information should be handled, who should have access to the information, and under what conditions the information should be disclosed.[95]

Interestingly, both preambles leave largely implicit the distinctions between HIPs and other professions *within* the health care arena (including both clinicians and administrators). Presumably, though, the core difference lies in the HIP's particular solicitude for information—its security, integrity, accuracy, usability, accessibility, and so on. This solicitude for information becomes more readily apparent in the bodies of the codes themselves, where calls for sound data-management are sometimes only loosely linked to specific human beneficiaries. AHIMA enunciates an obligation to "preserve, protect, and secure personal health information in any form or medium and hold in the highest regard the contents of the records."[96] IMIA invokes seven "General Principles of Informatic Ethics," including "openness," "security," and "access,"[97] and from these it derives (among other things) a duty "to ensure that appropriate measures are in place . . . to safeguard the (a) security, (b) integrity, (c) material quality, (d) usability, and (e) accessibility of electronic records."[98] To understand the distinctive ethical position of a HIP in the health care workplace, one need only ponder how many clinicians or health care administrators would see themselves as having a free-standing duty—independent of patient health or organizational efficiency—to protect the transparency of record-keeping procedures and the accessibility of records.

At the same time, the IMIA and AHIMA codes are not simply reducible to the generic ethics of responsible data-management. Formally, at least, both codes place top priority on the HIP's duties to the patient, and within those, on traditional medical-ethics issues of (a) patient awareness, consent, and self-determination; and (b) medical-record privacy, confidentiality, and non-intrusiveness. Both codes also highlight duties of teamwork and collegiality toward other health care professionals, and duties to serve as an IT educator and advocate not only in the workplace but also in public forums. The IMIA code adds a detailed list of "good employee" duties toward the HIP's employing entity,[99] while the AHIMA code places somewhat more emphasis on "good citizenship" duties toward the profession and the public—including a duty to participate in "[pro-bono] activities that promote respect for the . . . profession,"[100] a duty to "contribute to the knowledge base of health information management,"[101] and, strikingly, a duty to "engage in social and political action that supports the protection of privacy."[102] On a more mundane level, the AHIMA code also enumerates a short list of illustrative HIP sins,[103] such as condoning retrospective catch-up documentation, up-coding clinical records to increase billings, hiding or ignoring unflattering performance data, misrepresenting information for physician credentialing or facility accreditation, covering up flawed or incomplete records, and misusing confidential or proprietary information. Although not comprehensive, this inventory gives a sense of the practical pressures and temptations that give HIP ethics a real-world relevance.

Taken as a whole, then, HIP ethics meld the librarian's commitment to systematicity and documentation; the computer scientist's commitment to integration, standardization, and reliability; and the clinician's commitment to health, beneficence, and consent. Although the relative priority of these sometimes competing commitments may vary from setting to setting and from practitioner to practitioner, the unique juxtaposition of desiderata sets HIPs apart from each of the kindred occupations that abut the health-information domain. In HIP ethics, we can see both a tacit jurisdictional claim and the germs of a distinctive professional world view.

Credentialing and Enclosure

Although a shared identity and a legitimating narrative are important accomplishments for any professional project, many accounts of professionalization—including some from the functionalist camp as well as virtually all from the critical camp—would reserve the label "profession" for the handful of occupations that manage to parlay their capacity for collective action and their aura of expert authority into an effective monopoly on work within their chosen jurisdiction. Thus, a final important indicator of HIP professionalization is the degree to which the emerging profession can exert influence over the market for its services. One step along this path is the establishment of widely recognized credentials for those who profess mastery of the profession's particular knowledge base. As can be seen in table 8.4, two associations lead the way in this area: AAPC offers both general and specialty credentials for coders (the CPC, CPC-H, CPC-P, and CIRCC), while AHIMA offers not only coder credentials (the CCA, CCS, and CCS-P) but also credentials for health information technicians (RHIT) and health information administrators (RHIA).[104] In recent years, AHIMA has instituted two additional specialty credentials, the first in health privacy and security (CHPS), and the second in health data analysis (CHDA), and HIMSS has joined the mix with a generalist credential of its own, the CPHIMS.[105]

Table 8.4   **HIP Credentials**

Sponsor	Credential	Acronym	Inception	Holders
AAPC	Certified Professional Coder	CPC	1988	55,000
	Certified Professional Coder – Hospital	CPC-H	1991	3,000
	Certified Professional Coder – Payer	CPC-P	2005	1,000
	Certified Interventional Radiology Cardiovascular Coder	CIRCC	2008	(new)
AHIMA	Registered Health Information Administrator	RHIA	1932	15,345
	Registered Health Information Technician	RHIT	1955	27,394
	Certified Coding Specialist	CCS	1992	9,760
	Certified Coding Specialist – Physician-based	CCS-P	1997	4,321
	Certified Coding Associate	CCA	2002	4,231
	Certified in Healthcare Privacy and Security	CHPS	2002	390
	Certified Health Data Analyst	CHDA	2008	(new)
HIMSS	Certified Professional in Healthcare Information and Management Systems	CPHIMS	2001	851

Despite the plethora of available credentials, the leading HIP associations have broadly similar certification requirements for each skill level.[106] To acquire a coding credential, a candidate typically must pass an examination sponsored by the granting organization. For both AAPC and AHIMA, these coder examinations consist of questions about the correct application of various standardized procedure, supply, and diagnosis coding schemes. AHIMA also requires a high school diploma and recommends some on-the-job training, while AAPC recommends an associate degree and requires membership in the association. For its RHIT and RHIA credentials (see table 8.4), AHIMA requires a degree from a CAHIIM-accredited training program, either at the associate level for the RHIT or at the baccalaureate level for the RHIA. In addition, RHIT and RHIA candidates must pass an examination that tests knowledge not only of coding basics such as health data standards and clinical classification systems, but also of reimbursement methodologies, health care statistics and research, security and privacy standards, and health care-related information and communication technologies. HIMSS's CPHIMS credential requires a similar examination, but raises the training criteria to demand either a baccalaureate degree plus five years of experience in information and management systems (at least three of those years in health care) or a graduate degree plus three years of experience (at least two of those in health care). On top of these entry requirements, all the major HIP certifications require continuing education to preserve the credential holder's good standing.

The accreditation of training programs is itself another indication of market influence. From 1943 until 2004, AHIMA accredited specialized programs in health informatics and information management, first in collaboration with the American Medical Association and then in collaboration with the Commission on Accreditation of Allied Health Education Programs. As mentioned above, this role has now passed to CAHIIM, which currently accredits approximately 250 different degree programs in health information management at the associate and baccalaureate levels. To become accredited, a candidate program must, among other things, meet or exceed the standards of AHIMA's Model Curriculum for Health Information Management.[107] At both the associate degree and baccalaureate levels, this curriculum requires general education courses and a practicum experience, as well as HIP-specific coursework covering: health data structures and standards; clinical classification systems; biomedical sciences; health care statistics and biomedical research methods; quality management; health services organization and delivery; health-information ethics and law; information technology and applied informatics; and organizational, financial, operations, and human resources management and planning.[108]

Of course, what matters critically for professional control over the HIP labor market is not the mere existence of credentials and accreditations, but the institutionalization of those credentials as "taken for granted" qualifications for work in the field. Here, the available evidence suggests that professionalization has exerted a tangible but limited impact on the market. For instance, AAPC's own analysis of its 2008 Salary Survey concluded, "Certification is still optional for many. Certification is required for only half of us in our current jobs; however, up from the 42 percent reported in the 2007 survey."[109] In addition, although the survey found that credentialed coders earned an average of $43,100 per year, compared to $36,500 for non-credentialed coders, the accompanying analysis suggested that most of this 18 percent gap could be explained by factors other than credentialing—such as type or size of employer, amount of training, geographical location, and the complexity of the coding being done. AHIMA's 2002 member survey yielded somewhat stronger results: nearly 60 percent of respondents reported that HIM positions in their workplaces were usually filled by HIM-credentialed professionals, and this figure rose to over 80 percent in consulting firms, educational institutions, and professional associations.[110] Indeed, 52 percent of RHIAs, 49 percent of RHITs, and 32 percent of CCSs and CCS-Ps reported that HIM credentials were "required" in their workplaces, compared to less than 5 percent of each group reporting that such credentials were "unnecessary or irrelevant." Further, only 13 percent of respondents said that credentials were unimportant for securing their current jobs, and only 16 percent believed that credentials were unimportant for advancement. Nonetheless, only 22.2 percent reported that HIM credentials were actually *required* for advancement.[111]

To get another perspective on the importance of credentials, one can examine postings on popular job-search Web sites. For the months of July, September, and October 2007, we systematically culled information from the Web site Monster.com, which maintains separate databases of job openings and job-seekers. Using the category "Medical Records, Health IT, and Informatics" as an approximation for the HIP labor market, we recorded the proportion of job listings and résumé postings that mentioned the following HIP credentials: RHIA, RHIT, CCA, CCS, CCS-P, CHPS, CPC, CPC-H, or CPC-P. Over these three months, 24 percent of the 4,593 job listings mentioned one or more of these credentials, while only 3.3 percent of the 58,831 résumé postings did the same. These admittedly rudimentary results can support competing interpretations: a 24 percent penetration of the workplace is a substantial but hardly overwhelming level of institutionalization; and a 3 percent penetration of the labor pools suggests that, whatever employers may think of HIP credentials, certification has hardly acquired a "taken-for-granted" status among the workforce. Nonetheless, it is likely that the employee side of the picture is somewhat diluted by casual job seekers; and, percentages notwithstanding, the absolute number of credentialed résumés (1,955) substantially exceeds the number of credential-seeking jobs (1,120). Overall, the evidence suggests that HIP credentials are gradually gaining a foothold in the labor market, but that credentialing has not yet become so pervasive or taken-for-granted as to be a de facto entry requirement.

Beyond credentialing as a market-signal, the Holy Grail for professional control over the market would be a formal de jure mandate reserving key parts of the HIP domain for licensed practitioners. To date, no segment of the health information field has achieved this milestone. While many states and the federal government work closely with the leading HIP associations on various policy initiatives, the profession's influence so far has been mostly normative and cognitive. Glimmers of formal legal backing may be starting to emerge, however: At the federal level, the Department of Health and Human Services' Office of Inspector General has issued a "guidance" encouraging hospitals to make sure that coding and audit personnel are "independent and qualified, *with the requisite certifications*" (emphasis added).[112] And at the state level, Hawaii's Insurance Code establishes a licensing regime for "independent [medical] bill reviewers" and waives the accompanying experience, training and examination requirements for any applicants who hold credentials from AAPC or AHIMA.[113]

Moreover, several HIP associations appear to be laying the groundwork for stronger, perhaps more regulative, state ties in the future. This trend is most visible in the role of HIP associations in formulating privacy and EDI standards under HIPAA: Although operating only in an advisory capacity, most of the major HIP associations contributed testimony and expertise during the legislative and regulatory phases of HIPAA's development, and aspects of the resulting rules (particularly the requirement that covered entities hire or designate a "privacy officer") seem tailor-made to further the HIP professional project. The trend toward HIP associations acquiring a quasi-regulative status can also be seen in the active support that AHIMA and HIMSS have provided to nascent IT-certification groups, such as the Certification Commission for Healthcare Information Technology (CCHIT), which develops criteria and inspection procedures for assessing the adequacy of electronic health record systems.[114] Such activities fall well short of an official state delegation of licensing, policymaking, or coercive authority to the emerging profession; nonetheless, they create precedents for state officials collaborating with—and, in the process, deferring to the judgments of—HIP associations on matters of substantial legal consequence.

HIPs in the System of Health Care Professions

HIPs So Far

In combination, the preceding observations portray a professional project that is well under way but still nascent. Health information workers have long been a fixture of the health care workplace, but both their numbers and their prominence have increased dramatically with the advent of the Internet, the passage of HIPAA and the push for an enhanced health information infrastructure. Medical records clerks have become health information technicians, IT directors have become CIOs, and computer-savvy care providers have become CMIOs and nursing informaticians. This process has occurred throughout the health care sector, but it has been most dramatic in tertiary-care hospitals, academic research centers, and other large institutions, where resources, visibility, public policy engagement, and economies of scale have combined to accelerate the shift toward clinical IT and toward "modern" information management.

As health information workers have become more numerous, more sophisticated and more prominent, they have also become more self-aware. Trade associations have grown and, more recently, begun to consolidate and specialize. Conferences have proliferated, and attendance numbers have ballooned. New journals have emerged, and existing journals have adjusted their missions to appeal to new pools of potential readers.

The efflorescence of conferences and journals also marks a quickening of cognitive and normative life in the field. As publications accumulate and training programs sprout across the academic terrain, the existence and relevance of a distinctive HIP knowledge base is becoming increasingly taken for granted. Moreover, this knowledge base is beginning to acquire moral as well as technical aspects: Spurred intellectually by developments in computer ethics, legally by the intercession of HIPAA, and organizationally by the treacherous crosscurrents of managed care, HIP leaders are advocating codes of practice, enunciating principled commitments, and encouraging policy activism as never before. In all these regards, professionalization seems indisputably to be afoot.

The path of this professional project, however, is not entirely free of potholes. Most obviously, the HIP field has yet to develop sufficient moral credibility and/or cognitive hegemony to engender widespread licensure requirements for HIP practitioners, legal mandates for a HIP imprimatur on IT decisions, or other state actions to enclose and protect the new profession's jurisdiction. Without these cornerstones of regulative institutionalization, the HIP field remains vulnerable to external challenges and incursions, whether from consumer-rights advocates, medical professionals, business managers, or public health authorities.

In reality, though, the absence of a state-sanctioned monopoly may be as much a symptom as a root cause of the HIP field's incomplete professionalization, and the greatest challenges for the HIP project may be both more diffuse and more subtle than a mere lack of legal endorsement. One fundamental challenge lies in the sheer heterogeneity of the HIP workforce, and in particular the large numbers of health information workers who possess only limited training, who exhibit only superficial engagement with the field's body of knowledge, and who perform relatively routine tasks with little discretion and at modest pay. To construct a set of professional structures that could span the gulf between the coders of AAPC and the CIOs of CHIME would be no small feat.

A second, equally substantial, challenge lies in the heterogeneity not of front-line HIP jobs but of field-level HIP institutions. As a matter of free-market ideology, the presence of six major HIP associations, offering a dozen credentials and directing students toward training programs in a half-dozen different fields, might seem like a good thing. But professions do not particularly thrive on unbridled market competition, and the proliferation of associations, journals, conferences, training programs, ethics codes, and credentials may ultimately forestall, not accelerate, progress toward professional taken-for-grantedness. Admittedly, organizational theory sometimes seems to imply that the legitimacy of a new endeavor will inevitably rise apace with increases in the number of participants;[115] but this may hold true primarily for rank-and-file participants such as producers in an industry, foot-soldiers in a social movement, and practitioners in a profession—not for field-level entities such as trade associations, academic disciplines, and accreditation bodies. To advance the professional project, such field-level actors must foster a coherent and comprehensible institutional order; and unfortunately, in the absence of strong coordination, a proliferation of "sense makers" may paradoxically make for less sense, not more.

HIPs to Come

What then might we expect of the HIP field in the future? As other chapters in this volume suggest, clinical IT has moved to the forefront of the health policy agenda, bringing with it a growing awareness of the complex governance challenges that clinical IT creates. More IT spending, more IT initiatives, more IT concerns, and more IT regulations all seem to favor the prospects of an emerging profession that can claim mastery not only over the technical difficulties of making health information work, but also over the ethical difficulties of making health information work for the greater good. Indeed, it is a truism of organizational theory that actors can gain power within an organization by asserting a capacity to manage and alleviate critical sources of uncertainty[116]—and as a corollary, that professionals can gain power by inflating the technical and institutional threats that emanate from their professed jurisdiction.[117] For all the reasons described above, the current health information terrain provides fertile ground for such professional self-aggrandizement: Clinical IT is, in itself, technically, economically, organizationally, politically, ethically, and legally uncertain, and any profession that can plausibly manage that uncertainty holds a powerful bargaining chip. But in addition, current IT trends—toward greater speed, greater volume, greater scope, greater integration, greater urgency, and greater legal sensitivity of clinical data flows—only serve to inflate the profession's ability to inflate the threat. Under these conditions, it seems hard to imagine that the coming years will be anything but expansionary ones for the HIP field.

Yet, if the preceding pages are correct, the HIP professional project may be approaching a crossroads. No matter how favorable the policy climate, the field's leaders may soon face difficult decisions about how to draw the profession's boundaries, how to structure the relationship between low-end and high-end workers, and how to allocate the ongoing labor (and the ongoing rewards) of maintaining, guiding, representing, and reproducing the profession as a whole. Research on institutional change suggests that this may be a fairly common stage for many new institutions, including many new professions, but it nonetheless marks a potentially perilous passage.[118]

There is no way to predict with any certainty how events in the sector will play out, but some paths seem more likely than others. It seems likely, for example, that the field has achieved sufficient "escape velocity" to separate itself from competing professions such as medicine and nursing, computer science, library science, and health care administration. Already, in conference programs, in academic curricula, and in codes of ethics, one can see the hammering out of coherent narratives that explain why health-information work is, at once: crucial to health but different from clinical care; central to technology implementation but different from IT development; essential for making health information usable but different from archive curation; and critical for effective and efficient health care enterprises but different from business administration. All of those boundaries may occasionally be challenged and traversed, but they seem unlikely to be erased in the foreseeable future.

As external jurisdictional boundaries become more secure, however, internal status tensions may become more salient. It seems unlikely, for example, that a single profession will be able to incorporate both the low and the high ends of the HIP continuum in a stable and collegial way; rather, one might expect further professionalization among technologists, information managers, and informaticians, at the high end, to be coupled with (and to some degree contingent upon) the solidification of a subordinate paraprofessional status for coders and information technicians, at the low end. Although it is hard to imagine even high-end HIPs ever acquiring quite the status and discretion of the classic "autonomous professions" of medicine and law,[119] one can more easily envision a future in which high-end HIPs would achieve a position akin to that of accountants: credentialed, respected for their expertise, identified with a distinctive outlook and character, and mandated by law for certain ethically sensitive tasks; yet almost as frequently employed in internal administrative roles within large bureaucracies as in freestanding professional partnerships and consulting firms.

These developments, if they transpire, would create both challenges and opportunities for the leading HIP associations. AHIMA, in particular, may eventually find itself forced to decide whether to continue the big-tent approach that has so far facilitated its growth, or whether instead to reframe its mission along the lines of more traditional professional bodies like the American Medical Association and the American Bar Aassociation. If AHIMA does ultimately choose to limit its core constituency to high-end health information professionals, AAPC would seem to be the obvious beneficiary, becoming the primary organizational representative—and quite likely the primary credentialing body—for the field's immense supporting cast of low-end paraprofessionals. This may not be a particularly glamorous role; but in a field where the low end outnumbers the high by almost 2.5 to 1, it is certainly a viable niche. AMIA, for its part, seems well positioned to be the field's intellectual leader, focusing on theoretical, philosophical, and educational issues (perhaps in collaboration with CAHIIM), while leaving the mundane political, economic, and organizational interests of workaday HIP practitioners largely to the ministrations of others. HIMSS's role in this scenario is less clear, in part because the organization seems increasingly focused on the needs of the health IT *industry* rather than on the needs of health information professionals qua professionals. This distinction may be slight, especially in an expansionary era; but despite the recent creation of the CPHIMS credential, it seems unlikely that HIMSS will effectively challenge AHIMA or AMIA for leadership of the HIP professional project. Rather, HIMSS seems well positioned to become a trade organization akin to the AHA, advocating for the sector but not playing a central role in the professionalization of the workforce. Finally, CHIME and AMDIS seem likely to remain what they are today: supplementary convening points for individuals whose interstitial roles (between HIPs and management, and between HIPs and clinicians, respectively) create distinctive perspectives, problems, and interests that are not fully addressed by the generalist professional associations at the field's core.

HIP Professionalization and Medical Professionalism

These speculations return us to the question that links the present chapter to the rest of this anthology: What role might the emerging health information professions play in mediating the impact of information technology on the professionalism of physicians, nurses, and other established groups within the health care field? Health care organizations are complex polities, and introducing a new professional claimant into the mix will undoubtedly affect the jurisdictions, capacities, and prerogatives of the other players; but where, exactly, the lines of allegiance and antagonism will fall remains unclear.

Certain affinities between the health information professions and the traditional medical professions are apparent: As part of the legacy of their separation from computer science and non-medical informatics, HIPs tend to have a strong commitment to the special character of *health* information, and solicitude for the particular vulnerabilities and concerns of patients. In this, they resemble health care practitioners, perhaps more than they resemble the business-oriented MBAs who now run many large health care systems. HIP ethics, like medical ethics, also place a high premium on the confidentiality of clinical information. HIPs may be more concerned about the unauthorized disclosure of that information beyond the perimeters of the information management system than about threats to the sacrosanct covenant of the doctor-patient relationship; but HIPs are likely to share clinicians' sense that third-party intrusions into the clinical record system fundamentally affront professional responsibility. Finally, HIPs in principle (although not always in practice) embrace an ethic of teamwork and participatory-design that takes the distinctive challenges of technology implementation seriously, and that balks at the covert or coercive imposition of information systems on unwilling or unwitting users. All these affinities make HIPs and clinicians likely allies in the face of pressures from "the business side" to exploit health information for marketing, commercial data-mining, price discrimination, and/or workplace surveillance. In these regards, HIPs may help to make medical practice in the new information age more professional, not less.

On the other hand, HIPs also have a strong commitment to the power of information, and to the gathering, management, aggregation, and use of information in ways that would maximize that power. In this, they resemble administrators (and public health officials), perhaps more than they resemble the front-line clinicians who still largely care for patients one case at a time. HIP ethics, like business ethics, also place a high premium on efficiency, order, security, and control, and most HIP ethical codes explicitly acknowledge that the information rights of individuals must sometimes be balanced against the information needs of groups—arguably including the administrative needs of health care organizations and the public health needs of the state. Further, because they bear day-to-day responsibility for making information systems work, HIPs have both a principled ethical investment and an immediate practical stake in the integrity of record-keeping practices, the security of computing networks, and the sanctity of data; and this protective impulse often overrides more pro-social principles of patient self-determination, participatory design, and user-friendliness. In many situations, these orientations are more likely to align HIPs with hospital administrators and public-health authorities than with clinicians, putting HIP professionalism and medical professionalism at least somewhat at odds.

Our research on HIPAA compliance and clinical IT implementation has revealed a number of contexts in which these inter-professional tensions surface.[120] One mundane source of friction centers on security measures like passwords and timeouts: Busy clinicians have trouble understanding why passwords must be arcane, frequently changed, and repeatedly reentered, and so their sense of professionalism as caregivers leads them to share log-ins with co-workers, scribble passwords on Post-it notes, and retrospectively update records during off-peak hours when there is less chance of being called away and timed out. HIPs, in contrast, have trouble understanding how anyone could be so cavalier about system integrity, and so their sense of professionalism as information managers leads them to push for sanctioning authority and to develop "technical safeguards" that are ever harder to circumvent and that are therefore all the more clinically intrusive.

Another, more dramatic, sore point involves "shadow charts"—duplicate patient records that clinicians maintain (usually in hard copy) in a ready location such as a desk-side filing drawer. For the clinician, the shadow chart is a harmless convenience in most cases, a safeguard against retrieval delays in some cases, and a device for keeping particularly sensitive patient information out of the inter-organizational data stream in at least a few cases. For the HIP, in contrast, the shadow chart is a fundamental threat to the integrity of the entire clinical record system: shadow charts spawn delays and omissions in updating the official file, thereby putting patients at risk; and shadow charts frustrate "professional" information management practices (and violate HIPAA requirements) for secure data storage and rigorous access accounting, thereby putting the organization at risk. In some hospitals, this struggle over shadow charts has esca-lated to the point where health information managers and privacy officers rou-tinely conduct "night raids" of physicians' offices, in search of contraband files.

Beyond these discreet dust-ups, HIPs and clinicians in many settings find themselves embroiled in much larger philosophical debates over the design, implementation, and use of multi-million-dollar clinical IT systems. To reap the maximum benefit from these systems, the HIP world view prescribes that use should be universal and non-optional, and that users should be encouraged—through technical constraints, through persuasion, and through sanctions if necessary—to employ standardized data fields whenever possible, and to min-imize reliance on verbal explanations and free-form notes. Clinicians, in con-trast, generally prize the nuances and flexibilities of open-ended charting, and resist efforts to reduce clinical details to a series of rigid check-boxes. Structured data-entry may be the only practical way to harness the power of clinical IT for systemic improvement, but systemic improvement is often a value closer to the hearts of administrators, policymakers, and the HIPs who serve them than to the hearts of front-line clinical caregivers.

Although each of these confrontations has its own idiosyncratic contours and its own colorful vocabulary of moves and countermoves, heroes and vil-lains, these encounters are not merely petty jurisdictional squabbles. Rather, they reflect genuine tensions between the competing values embedded in any clinical IT system—tensions that would exist (in latency at least) even if there were no cadre of HIPs to bring them to the fore. Nonetheless, the emergence of HIPs as champions of some of these values over others means that the course of medical professionalism in the new information age will depend not only on the medical profession's own assessment of what constitutes sound and ethical IT use, but also on the inter-professional balance of power in particular sites of practice. The importance of HIPs, then, may lie less in their potential for trans-forming health IT per se, than in their potential for transforming the surround-ing politics of the health care workplace.

Conclusion

The arc of this chapter began with theory, passed through evidence, and ended with speculation. It seems clear that a professional project in the health infor-mation domain is, indeed, under way. It also seems clear that this project is approaching—or perhaps has already passed—the point of no return. Certainly, nothing in current health policy debates suggests a diminished role for HIPs in the future. Indeed, much to the contrary, the demand for professional health information management is likely to rise dramatically as the new health information infrastructure unfolds and as its power becomes apparent. Moreover, even the concerns of health IT's detractors seem unlikely to forestall the rise of HIPs—for, unless a wave of precautionary fervor quashes health IT entirely, warnings of health IT's dangers seem likely to augment, not reduce, the demand for informed, ethical and accountable professionals to guide IT use. This has been the experience of HIPAA, and it is likely to be the experience of future IT initiatives as well. HIPs are here, and they are probably here to stay.

What remains to be seen is whether HIPs, in their growing influence, will become allies or adversaries of the traditional clinical professions and of traditional clinical professionalism. HIPs could easily join with health care practitioners to embrace the distinctive responsibilities of the clinical encounter and to defend the boundary between the health care vocation of "*health* information management" and the commercial vocation of "*management* information systems." But HIPs could equally easily join with health care managers to embrace the economic imperatives of rationality and control, and to defend the boundary between the systemic vocation of "health information *management*" and the pastoral vocation of "*clinical* medicine." Given the pace of recent developments, we may not need to wait long for an answer. But anyone who cares about the fate of medical professionalism in the new information age should have ample reason to care about the fate of health information professionalism as well.

Notes

Chapter 1. Expecting the Unexpected

1. In proton beam therapy a cyclotron accelerates subatomic particles down a lead-shielded tunnel the length of a football field before they slam into patients' tumors.
2. Catherine DesRoches, Eric G. Campbell, S. R. Rao, K. Donelan, Timothy G. Ferris et al. "Electronic Health Records in Ambulatory Care: A National Survey of Physicians," *New England Journal of Medicine* 359, no. 1 (July 3, 2008): 50–60.
3. Ashish K. Jha, Timothy G. Ferris, K. Donelan, Catherine DesRoches, A.Shields et al., "How Common Are Electronic Health Records in the United States? A Summary of the Evidence," *Health Affairs (Millwood)* 25 (2006): w496–w507.
4. Julia Adler-Milstein, A. P. McAfee, D. W. Bates, Ashish K. Jha, "The State of Regional Health Information Organizations: Current Activities and Financing," *Health Affairs (Millwood)* 27 (2008): w60–w69.
5. Denis Protti, G. Wright, S. Treweek, and I. Johansen, "Primary Care Computing in England and Scotland: A Comparison with Denmark," *Inform Primary Care* 14 (2006): 93–99.

Chapter 2. Quality Regulation in the Information Age

1. See, for example, Linda T. Kohn, Janet M. Corrigan, and Molla S. Donaldson, eds., *To Err Is Human: Building a Safer Health System* (Washington, DC: National Academy Press, 2000); Institute of Medicine, *Crossing the Quality Chasm: A New Health System for the 21st Century* (Washington, DC: National Academy Press, 2001); Elizabeth A. McGlynn, S. M. Asch, J. Adams, J. Keesey, J. Hicks, et al., "The Quality of Health Care Delivered to Adults in the United States," *New England Journal of Medicine* 348, no. 26 (June 26, 2003): 2635–2645.
2. See American Board of Internal Medicine Foundation, American College of Physicians–American Society of Internal Medicine Foundation, and European Federation of Internal Medicine, "Medical Professionalism in the New Millennium: A Physician Charter," *Annals of Internal Medicine* 136, no. 3 (February 5, 2002): 243–246 (hereafter "Physician Charter") (identifying primacy of patient welfare, patient autonomy, and social justice as three "fundamental principles" of professionalism).
3. For a more comprehensive discussion of health care quality regulation in the aftermath of the information revolution, see Kristin Madison, "Health Care Quality Regulation in an Information Age," *U.C. Davis Law Review* 40, no. 5 (2007): 1577–1652, upon which this chapter's discussion of regulation draws heavily.
4. Michelle Mello, Carly Kelly, and Troyen Brennan have also defined regulation broadly, "to include any organized and deliberate leveraging of power or authority to effect changes in the behavior of health care providers." Michelle Mello, Carly Kelly, and Troyen Brennan, "Fostering Rational Regulation of Patient Safety," *Journal of Health Politics, Policy and Law* 30, no. 3 (2005): 376.
5. This schema resembles, but differs in important ways from, other schema used to classify market and regulatory mechanisms in health care. See, for instance, Clark C. Havighurst, "The Professional Paradigm of Medical Care: Obstacle to Decentralization," *Jurimetrics Journal* 30, no. 4 (1990): 415–430; Einer R. Elhauge, "Can Health Law

Become a Coherent Field of Law?" *Wake Forest Law Review* 41, no. 2 (2006): 365–390.

6. See generally, Arnold M. Epstein, Thomas H. Lee, and Mary Beth Hamel, "Paying Physicians for High-Quality Care," *New England Journal of Medicine* 350, no. 4 (January 22, 2004): 406–410 (describing pay-for-performance programs).

7. For a more thorough analysis of the effects of information technology-driven cost reductions on health care quality regulations, see Madison, "Health Care Quality Regulation," 1595–1603; see also Timothy Stoltzfus Jost, "Oversight of the Quality of Medical Care: Regulation, Management, or the Market?" *Arizona Law Review* 37, no. 3 (1995): 850–857 (describing how information technology promoted the expansion of health care report cards and total quality management programs).

8. The Agency for Healthcare Research and Quality has assembled a database on public and private health care reporting efforts. See U.S. Department of Health and Human Services, Agency for Healthcare Research and Quality, "Health Care Report Card Compendium," www.talkingquality.gov/compendium/.

9. See U.S. Department of Health and Human Services, "Hospital Compare," www.hospitalcompare.hhs.gov.

10. Pennsylvania Health Care Cost Containment Council ("PHC4"), *Pennsylvania's Guide to Coronary Artery Bypass Graft Surgery 2004* (February 2006), 2–5, www.phc4.0rg/reports/cabg/04/docs/cabg2004report.pdf; PHC4, *Total Hip and Knee Replacements* (June 2005), 7–23, www.phc4.0rg/reports/hipknee/02/docs/hipkneeFY2002report.pdf.

11. See New York State Department of Health, "New York State Hospital Profile," hospitals.nyhealth.gov; New Jersey Department of Health and Senior Services, *Hospital Performance Report: A Consumer Report* (2008), http://web.doh.state.nj.us/hpr/docs/2008/report.pdf; Texas Department of State Health Services, "Indicators of Inpatient Care in Texas Hospitals, 2004, Hospital Database," www.dshs.state.tx.us/THCIC/Publications/Hospitals/IQIReport2004/IQIReport2004.shtm.

12. Florida Agency for Health Care Administration, "Agency for Health Care Administration Announces the Launch of Florida Compare Care," press release, November 8, 2005, http://ahca.myflorida.com/SCHS/pdf/comparecarecebsiterollout_11–08.pdf; Florida Agency for Health Care Administration, FloridaHealthFinder.Gov, "Hospitals and Ambulatory Surgery Centers," www.floridahealthfinder.gov/CompareCare/SelectChoice.aspx.

13. Colorado Hospital Report Card Act, Colorado Revised Statutes, sec. 25–3–701 (Bradford 2006); Governor Bill Owens, "Owens Signs Health Care Bills," press release, June 2, 2006, http://web.archive.org/web/20060608005027/http://www.colorado.gov/governor/press/june06/healthcare.html.

14. See Governor Matt Blunt, "Blunt Aims to Protect Patients from Healthcare-Associated Infections," press release, December 28, 2006; Missouri Department of Health and Senior Services, "Missouri Healthcare-Associated Infection Reporting," www.dhss.mo.gov/HAI/.

15. See PHC4, "Pennsylvania Releases Nation's First Hospital-Specific Report on Hospital-Acquired Infections," press release, November 14, 2006, www.phc4.0rg/reports/hai/05/nr111406.htm; PHC4, "Hospital-Acquired Infections in Pennsylvania," www.phc4.0rg/hai/Default.aspx.

16. Joint Commission, "Quality Check," www.qualitycheck.org/.

17. See Leapfrog Group, "What Does Leapfrog Ask Hospitals?" www.leapfroggroup.org/for_consumers/hospitals_asked_what (accessed January 14, 2009).

18. See California HealthCare Foundation, "About Us," www.calhospitalcompare .org/About-Us.aspx (describing participants in report card development) (accessed January 14, 2009).

19. See, for example, Independence Blue Cross, "HealthGrades Physician and Hospital Quality Guides," www.ibx.com/members/health_resources/healthgrades.html (explaining that its Web site includes HealthGrades-supplied information on physician education, training, licensure, board certification, and medical board disciplinary actions, among other measures) (accessed January 14, 2009).

20. See Massachusetts Board of Registration in Medicine, "On-Line Physician Profile Site," profiles.massmedboard.org/MA-Physician-Profile-Find-Doctor.asp; see also Frances H. Miller, "Illuminating Patient Choice: Releasing Physician-Specific Data to the Public," *Loyola Consumer Law Reporter* 8, no. 2 (1996): 125 (describing origins of the Massachusetts Web site).

21. See, for example, Maryland Board of Physicians, "Practitioner Profile System," www.mbp.state.md.us/bpqapp/; Medical Board of California, "Physician License Lookup," www.medbd.ca.gov/lookup.htm1; Minnesota Board of Medical Practice, "Health Professional Database," www.docboard.org/mn/df/mndf.htm.

22. See PHC4, "Cardiac Surgery in Pennsylvania 2006 Hospital Data," www.phc4 .org/cabg/ (accessed January 14, 2009); New York State Department of Health, "Adult Cardiac Surgery in New York State, 2002–2004" (2006), www.health .state.ny.us/diseases/cardiovascular/heart_disease/docs/cabg_2002–2004.pdf.

23. See California Office of the Patient Advocate, "Medical Group Ratings," www.opa .ca.gov/report_card/medicalgroupcounty.aspx.

24. See Massachusetts Health Quality Partners (MHQP), "Home," www.mhqp.org.

25. Health plans' use of performance measurement has proved controversial. Recently, a number of insurers have taken steps to improve transparency in the rating process. In 2007, under settlement agreements with the New York Attorney General, several health insurers committed to adopting measures designed to ensure accuracy, transparency, and oversight of the measurement process. See, for example, Attorney General Andrew M. Cuomo, "Attorney General Cuomo Announces Agreement with CIGNA Creating a New National Model for Doctor Ranking Programs," press release, October 29, 2007, http://www.oag.state.ny.us/media_center/2007/oct/oct29a_07 .html. In 2008, a number of health insurers agreed to a similar set of transparency principles. See Consumer-Purchaser Disclosure Project, "Consumers, Health Care Purchasers, Physicians, and Health Insurers Announce Agreement on Principles to Guide Physician Performance Rating," press release, April 1, 2008, http:// healthcaredisclosure.org/docs/files/PatientCharterDisclosureRelease040108.pdf.

26. See U.S. Department of Health and Human Services, Centers for Medicare and Medicaid Services, "Physician Quality Reporting Initiative," www.cms.hhs .gov/PQRI (accessed January 14, 2009).

27. See Epstein, Lee, and Hamel, "Paying Physicians," 407–408 (describing the Bridges to Excellence program and providing examples of other pay-for-performance programs).

28. Ibid.

29. See Meredith B. Rosenthal, B. E. Landon, S. L. Normand, R. G. Frank, and A. M. Epstein, "Pay for Performance in Commercial HMOs," *New England Journal of Medicine* 355, no. 18 (November 2, 2006): 1895.

30. See Karen Llanos, Joanie Rothstein, Mary Beth Dyer and Michael Bailit, *Physician Pay-for-Performance in Medicaid: A Guide for States* (Center for Health Care Strategies, 2007), www.chcs.org/usr_doc/Physician_P4P_Guide.pdf.

31. See Centers for Medicare and Medicaid Services, "Medicare 'Pay for Performance (P4P)' Initiatives," press release, January 31, 2005, www.cms.hhs.gov/apps/media/press/release.asp?Counter=1343.

32. See Karen Milgate and Sharon Bee Cheng, "Pay-for-Performance: The MedPAC Perspective," *Health Affairs (Millwood)* 25, no. 2 (2006): 413.

33. See Department of Health and Human Services, Centers for Medicare and Medicaid Services, "Medicare Program; Changes to the Hospital Inpatient Prospective Payment Systems and Fiscal Year 2008 Rates; Final Rule," *Federal Register* 72, no. 162 (August 22, 2007): 47, 200.

34. A recent study on professionalism in medicine documents widespread physician agreement with the charter's basic principles. Eric G. Campbell, S. Regan, R. L. Gruen, Timothy G. Ferris, S. D. Rao, P. D. Cleary, and David Blumenthal, "Professionalism in Medicine: Results of a National Survey of Physicians," *Annals of Internal Medicine* 147, no. 11 (December 11, 2007): 795–802.

35. See "Physician Charter," 244.

36. See ibid., 245.

37. One aspect of professionalism is professional autonomy, which means that physicians are free, by and large, to choose their patients as they see fit. This freedom to turn away less desirable patients is not articulated in the high-aspiring Physician Charter, but it has been a basic aspect of other professional codes throughout time. The American Medical Association's Principles of Medical Ethics, for instance, has said since 1923 that "a physician shall . . . be free to choose whom to service," except in emergencies. See http://www.ama-assn.org/ama/pub/physician-resources/medical-ethics/code-medical-ethics/history-ama-ethics.shtml.

38. See, for example, Rachel M. Werner and David A. Asch, "The Unintended Consequences of Publicly Reporting Quality Information," *Journal of the American Medical Association* 293, no. 10 (March 9, 2005): 1239 (explaining that public reporting "may have unintended and negative consequences on health care" such as encouraging physicians to avoid especially sick patients or engage in inappropriate interventions in order to improve quality ratings); compare Nathan A. Bostick, Robert M. Sade, and John W. McMahon, Sr., "Report of the Council on Ethical and Judicial Affairs: Physician Pay-for-Performance," *Indiana Health Law Review* 3, no. 2 (2006): 435–436 (noting that pay-for-performance incentives may discourage physicians from serving vulnerable patient populations).

39. See Ronald M. Davis, "Autonomy v. Accountability: A Delicate Balance," *American Medical News* 50, no. 31 (August 20, 2007): 25, http://www.ama-assn.org/amednews/2007/08/20/edca0820.htm.

40. Ibid.

41. See Jost, "Oversight of the Quality of Medical Care," 864–865 (advocating use of practice pattern information to identify underperforming physicians).

42. See American Board of Internal Medicine, "Self-Evaluation of Practice Performance," www.abim.org/moc/mocsepp.aspx (accessed January 14, 2009) (describing quality measurement-related certification requirements).

43. See Catharine W. Burt, Esther Hing, and David Woodwell, "Electronic Medical Record Use by Office-Based Physicians: United States, 2005," www.cdc.gov/nchs/products/pubs/pubd/hestats/electronic/electronic.htm.

44. Compare Jordan J. Cohen, Sylvia Cruess, and Christopher Davidson, "Alliance Between Society and Medicine: The Public's Stake in Medical Professionalism," *Journal of the American Medical Association* 298, no. 6 (August 8, 2007): 670, 672

(arguing that a medical-societal alliance is needed to "establish the technological infrastructure and legal arrangements needed to . . . enable robust quality-improvement activities" and that "broad agreement on data standards to ensure interoperability and on privacy laws to ensure access to relevant patient information" is required).

45. See "Physician Charter," 244.

46. See ibid.

47. *Johnson v. Kokemoor*, 545 N.W.2d 495 (Wis. 1996).

48. See *Duttry v. Patterson*, 771 A.2d 1255, 1259 (Pa. 2001) (holding that informed consent law does not require a surgeon to disclose lack of experience with a particular cancer surgery, even though a patient claimed she asked the surgeon about his experience with the procedure); *Whiteside v. Lukson*, 947 P.2d 1263, 1265 (Wash. Ct. App. 1997) (holding that informed consent law does not require a surgeon to disclose lack of experience in performing a new type of gallbladder removal).

49. *Albany Urology Clinic, P.C. v. Cleveland*, 528 S.E.2d 777, 782 n.19 (Ga. 2000).

50. *Kaskie v. Wright*, 589 A.2d 213, 216–17 (Pa. Super. Ct. 1991).

51. *Whiteside*, 947 P.2d at 1265.

52. *Cleveland*, 528 S.E.2d at 782 n.19.

53. Ibid.

54. *Ehlmann v. Kaiser Foundation Health Plan*, 198 F.3d 552, 558 (5th Cir. 2000) (rejecting fiduciary claim under ERISA); *Neade v. Portes*, 739 N.E.2d 496, 506 (Ill. 2000) (rejecting fiduciary claim under state law).

55. Mark A. Hall, "The Theory and Practice of Disclosing HMO Physician Incentives," *Law and Contemporary Problems* 65, no. 4 (Autumn 2002): 207–240.

56. *Arato v. Avedon*, 858 P.2d 598, 606 (Cal. 1993).

57. See "Physician Charter," 244.

58. See ibid., 245.

59. See ibid.

60. For more discussion of the effects of the different regulatory approaches, see Madison, "Health Care Quality Regulation," 1614–1624.

61. Note, however, that if care above the minimum quality threshold is more costly than care below it, a minimum threshold might reduce access to care for those with limited financial resources.

62. Research suggests that physicians perceive members of racial minorities to be less likely to follow treatment recommendations. See Rachel M. Werner, David A. Asch, and Daniel Polsky, "Racial Profiling: The Unintended Consequences of Coronary Artery Bypass Graft Report Cards," *Circulation* 111, no. 10 (March 15, 2005): 1262, and the sources cited therein (describing studies on physician perceptions of minority patients).

63. See Lawrence P. Casalino, A. Elster, A. Eisenberg, E. Lewis, J. Montgomery, and D. Ramos, "Will Pay-for-Performance and Quality Reporting Affect Health Care Disparities?" *Health Affairs (Millwood)* 26, no. 3 (April 10, 2007): w407 (suggesting that physicians might avoid patients who are members of racial minorities based on their perception that these patients will be less likely to comply with treatment recommendations and more likely to have poor outcomes). See also ibid., w408 (discussing studies showing links between report card results and patient characteristics such as health status, language, and socioeconomic status).

64. See David Dranove, D. Kessler, M. McClellan, and M. Satterthwaite, "Is More Information Better? The Effects of Report Cards on Health Care Providers," *Journal of Political Economy* 111, no. 3 (2003): 583–584 (reporting evidence of report card–related changes in provider selection of patients).

65. See Werner, Asch, and Polsky, "Racial Profiling," 1262.
66. Compare Bostick, Sade, and McMahon, "Physician Pay for Performance," 436 (noting that "[p]racticing physicians can promote equitable access by continuing to treat patients on the basis of need," despite the contrary incentives of pay-for-performance programs).
67. Susannah Fox, *Online Health Search 2006* (Washington, DC: Pew Internet and American Life Project, 2006): i, www.pewinternet.org/pdfs/PIP_Online_Health _2006.pdf.
68. Kaiser Family Foundation and Agency for Healthcare Research and Quality, *2006 Update on Consumers' Views of Patient Safety and Quality Information* (September 2006): 4–5, www.kff.org/kaiserpolls/upload/7559.pdf.
69. For example, one article suggests that report cards may not serve vulnerable patient groups well, including "the poor, the less educated, the uninsured, the chronically sick, and members of minority ethnic and language groups." Huw T. O. Davies, A. Eugene Washington, and Andrew B. Bindman, "Health Care Report Cards: Implications for Vulnerable Patient Groups and the Organizations Providing Them Care," *Journal of Health Politics, Policy and Law* 27, no. 3 (2002): 380.
70. See, for example, William M. Sage, "Regulating through Information: Disclosure Laws and American Health Care," *Columbia Law Review* 99, no. 7 (1999): 1822 (observing that information technology-based disclosure regimes may increase disparities because of socioeconomic differences in technology availability and use).
71. See Pew Internet and American Life Project, Demographics of Internet Users, www.pewinternet.org/trends/User_Demo_1.11.07.htm (accessed January 14, 2009). For example, 33 percent of adult respondents over age sixty-five were Internet users, as compared to over 80 percent of those under fifty; 54 percent of those making less than $30,000 per year were Internet users, as compared to 94 percent of those with incomes over $75,000; and 38 percent of those with less than high school education were Internet users, as compared to 92 percent who had completed college or graduate degrees. Ibid. Another survey suggests that the young are more likely to use information on the quality of health care than the elderly; among the elderly, only 14 percent said that they would be very likely to go to a Web site for information on the quality of physicians, hospitals, or health plans, while 42 percent of those under sixty-five would. Kaiser Family Foundation and Agency for Healthcare Research and Quality, *2006, Update on Consumers' Views*, 14, www.kff.org/kaiserpolls/ upload/7559.pdf.
72. For example, 33 percent of Internet users aged thirty-nine to forty-nine used the Internet to search for information about a physician or hospital, as compared to 18 percent of those over sixty-five; 40 percent of Internet-user college graduates had used the Internet to search for physician information, as compared to 21 percent of high school-educated Internet users. See Susannah Fox, *Online Health Search 2006*, 4, www.pewinternet.org/pdfs/PIP_Online_Health_2006.pdf.
73. See, e.g., Jost, "Oversight of the Quality of Medical Care," 853–855 (describing limitations on consumers' ability to use health care report cards); Sage, "Regulating through Information," 1728–1731 (describing health literacy and rationality barriers to effective report card use); Casalino et al., "Will Pay for Performance," w405–w414 (explaining that the poorly educated may be less likely to benefit from report cards, potentially increasing disparities); Davies, Washington, and Bindman, "Health Care Report Cards," 379–399 (including the poorly educated among vulnerable groups potentially underserved by report cards).

74. See also Clark C. Havighurst and Barak D. Richman, "Who Pays? Who Benefits? Distributive Injustice(s) in American Health Care," *Law and Contemporary Problems* 69, no. 4 (Autumn 2006): 7 (analyzing this phenomenon more broadly throughout health care finance and regulation).

75. See, for example, Casalino et al., "Will Pay for Performance," w409–w411 (suggesting ways to redesign quality reporting and pay-for-performance programs to limit their effects on disparities, including rewarding quality improvement and disparity reduction, applying better risk adjustment techniques, and other approaches).

76. See Bostick, Sade, and McMahon, "Physician Pay for Performance," 436 (encouraging physicians designing pay-for-performance programs to avoid structures that would discourage treating members of vulnerable groups).

77. Compare Casalino et al., "Will Pay for Performance," w411 (proposing that reporting and pay-for-performance programs assess effects on disparities).

78. See William M. Sullivan, "Can Professionalism Still Be a Viable Ethic?" *The Good Society* 13, no. 1 (2004): 18; Cohen, Cruess, and Davidson, "Alliance between Society and Medicine," 673.

79. See generally, Jost, "Oversight of the Quality of Medical Care," 825–868 (describing how information technology supports managerial and market approaches to quality oversight).

80. See, for example, Davis, "Autonomy and Accountability," 25 (commenting on discussion at the American Medical Association's annual meeting opposing pay-for-performance and arguing for a balance between physician autonomy and accountability); Timothy G. Ferris, C. Vogeli, J. Marder, C. S. Sennett, and Eric G. Campbell, "Physician Specialty Societies and the Development of Physician Performance Measures," *Health Affairs (Millwood)* 26, no. 6 (2007): 1716 (describing some specialty society members' reluctance to adopt performance measures).

81. Physicians can help to identify and implement measures that address the concerns of minority populations, for example. See Davies, Washington, and Bindman, "Health Care Report Cards," 3383–3386 (arguing for creation of quality measures that reflect interests of vulnerable patient groups).

82. Contrast, for instance, sociologist Eliot Freidson's early work, *Professional Dominance: The Social Structure of Medical Care* (New York: Atherton Press, 1970) with his later work, *Professionalism, the Third Logic: On the Practice of Knowledge* (Chicago: University of Chicago Press, 2001).

83. Ferris et al., "Physician Specialty Societies," 1716.

84. See ibid., 1713 (mentioning limited expertise as a constraint on specialty society participation in measure development).

Chapter 3. The "Information Rx"

Acknowledgments: Research and writing of this chapter have been supported by the Robert Wood Johnson Foundation. I would like to thank the following people for helpful comments on earlier drafts: David Blumenthal, Eugene Declercq, Mark Hall, Marc A. Rodwin, Sara Rosenbaum, David J. Rothman, Sheila M. Rothman, and Christopher Sellers.

1. Quoted in "Doctors Getting Rated by Zagat," *Business Insurance*, October 29, 2007.

2. "Would You Like Dessert with Your Diagnosis?" *USA Today* January 17, 2008; "Doctors Getting Rated by Zagat"; James King, "Ratings Can Mislead," *USA Today*, January 17, 2008.

3. "Would You Like Dessert with Your Diagnosis?"

4. Arnold M. Epstein, "Cures for an Ailing System," *Newsweek*, December 10, 2007, 78–84, Online LexisNexis® Academic; Regina E. Herzlinger, *Market Driven Health Care: Who Wins, Who Loses in the Transformation of America's Largest Service Industry* (Cambridge, MA: Perseus Books, 1997); Herzlinger, *Who Killed Health Care?* (New York: McGraw-Hill, 2007); Michael L. Millenson, *Demanding Medical Excellence: Doctors and Accountability in the Information Age* (Chicago: University of Chicago Press, 1999). Millenson's book offers an excellent overview of the quality-assessment movement's development over the past twenty years.

5. Theodore Roszak, "Politics of Information and the Fate of the Earth," *Progressive Librarian* 6/7 (Winter/Spring 1993), 1. See also Roszak, *The Cult of Information*, 2nd ed. (Berkeley: University of California Press, 1994).

6. Mark Peterson, "The Congressional Graveyard for Health Care Reform," in *Healthy, Wealthy, and Fair: Health Care and the Good Society*, ed. James A. Morone and Lawrence R. Jacobs (New York: Oxford University Press, 2005), 206–233.

7. Wendy Espeland and Michael Sauder, "Rankings and Reactivity: How Public Measures Recreate Social Worlds," *American Journal of Sociology* 113, no. 1 (July 2007): 1–40; quote on 1. See also Sarah E. Igo, *The Averaged American: Surveys, Citizens, and the Making of a Mass Public* (Cambridge, MA: Harvard University Press, 2007). For broader attempts to historicize the concept of the "information revolution," see Daniel R. Headrick, *When Information Came of Age: Technologies of Knowledge in the Age of Reason and Revolution, 1700–1850* (New York: Oxford University Press, 2000) and Richard R. John, "Rendezvous with Information? Computers and Communications Networks in the United States," *Business History Review* 75, no. 1 (Spring 2001): 1–13.

8. Headrick, *When Information Came of Age*; Theodore M. Porter, *Trust in Numbers: The Pursuit of Objectivity in Science and Public Life* (Princeton: Princeton University Press, 1996).

9. On the report card, see David Tyack, *The One Best System: A History of American Urban Education* (Cambridge, MA: Harvard University Press, 1974). For its expanding uses in the interwar period, see, for example, J. T. Worlston, "Shall We Eliminate the Comparative Marking System from the Report Card?" *Elementary School Journal* 33, no. 3 (November 1932): 176–184.

10. For a typical invocation of Nightingale as an assessment pioneer, see Patrice L. Spath, "Nursing Performance Measures Go Public," *Outcomes Management for Nursing Practice* 2, no. 3 (July/Sept. 1998): 124–129. Note that in the 1990s when the term "report card" became popular, states renamed these vital statistics reports, which they had been issuing for decades, as "health report cards."

11. Kenneth Ludmerer, *Learning to Heal: The Development of American Medical Education* (New York: Basic Books, 1986), especially 166–190.

12. On Codman, see Susan M. Reverby, "Stealing the Golden Eggs: Ernest Amory Codman and the Science and Management of Medicine," *Bulletin of the History of Medicine* 55, no. 2 (Summer 1981): 156–171. Codman's epitaph quote is on 170. The end result system reflected what Codman described as "the common sense notion that every hospital should follow every patient it treats, long enough to determine whether or not the treatment has been successful, and then to inquire, if not, why not, with a view to preventing a similar failure in the future" (158). Like Nightingale, Codman is frequently cast as a pioneer of quality assessment. See, for example, Kathy A. Badger, "Patient Care Report Cards: An Analysis," *Outcomes Management for Nursing Practice* 2, no. 1 (Jan./Mar.1998): 29–36.

13. The JCAH was formed in 1951 by representatives of the American College of Surgeons, the American College of Physicians, the American Medical Association, the American Hospital Association, and the Canadian Medical Association. The CMA later left to form its own accrediting body. For a timeline of the Joint Commission's history, see http://www.jointcommission.org/AboutUs/joint _commission.history.htm.

14. I develop this argument at greater length in Nancy Tomes, "Patients or Health Care Consumers? Why the History of Contested Terms Matters," *History and Health Policy in the United States: Putting the Past Back In*, ed. Rosemary A. Stevens, Charles E. Rosenberg, and Lawton R. Burns (New Brunswick, NJ: Rutgers University Press, 2006), 83–110.

15. Harold Aaron, *Good Health and Bad Medicine* (New York: Robert McBride, 1940). My arguments here are drawn from Tomes, "Patients or Health Care Consumers?" and Nancy Tomes, "The 'Great American Medicine Show' Revisited," *Bulletin of the History of Medicine* 79, no. 4 (Winter 2005), 627–663.

16. Lisabeth Cohen, *A Consumers' Republic: The Politics of Mass Consumption in Postwar America* (New York: Knopf, 2003); Lawrence Glickman, "The Strike in the Temple of Consumption," *Journal of American History* 88, no. 1 (June 2001): 99–126.

17. Michael Pertschuk, *Giant Killers* (New York: W. W. Norton, 1986). See also Tomes, "Patients or Health Care Consumers?"

18. This example is drawn from Nancy Tomes, "Medicine Shop: The Making of the Modern Health Consumer," manuscript in preparation.

19. Howard Shapiro, *How To Keep Them Honest: Herbert Denenberg on Spotting the Professional Phonies, Unscrewing Insurance, and Protecting Your Interests* (Emmaus, PA: Rodale Press, 1974). The nickname "Horrible Herb" is mentioned on 4.

20. Pennsylvania Insurance Department, *Shopper's Guide to Hospitals in the Philadelphia Area* (Harrisburg, PA: Department of Insurance, 1971); Ralph Nader, *Unsafe at Any Speed: The Designed-in Dangers of the American Automobile* (New York: Grossman, 1965).

21. Pennsylvania Insurance Department, *Shopper's Guide*, 1.

22. Shapiro, *How to Keep Them Honest*, 7.

23. A good overview of these developments is provided in Millenson, *Demanding Medical Excellence.*

24. Avedis Donabedian, "Evaluating the Quality of Medical Care," *Milbank Memorial Fund Quarterly*, 44, no. 2 (July 1966): 166–203.

25. For a good discussion of the factors leading to the quality assessment movement, see Arnold M. Epstein, "The Role of Quality Measurement in a Competitive Marketplace," *Baxter Health Policy Review* 2 (1996): 207–234.

26. For a succinct summary of Wennberg's work, see Millenson, *Demanding Medical Excellence*, 43–49.

27. Paul M. Ellwood, "Outcomes Management: A Technology of Patient Experience," *Archives of Pathology and Laboratory Medicine* 121, no. 11 (Nov. 1997): 1137–1144; Nicholas A. Hanchak, "Managed Care, Accountability, and the Physician," *Medical Clinics of North America* 80, no. 2 (March 1996): 245–261.

28. Victor Cohn, "Behind the Hospital Death Statistics," *Washington Post*, December 22, 1987, Z7. The 1981 Institute of Medicine study is quoted in this article.

29. Ibid., and Robert Pear, "Mortality Data Released for 6,000 U.S. Hospitals," *New York Times*, December 18, 1987; Matt Clark and Bob Cohn, "Sickbeds and Deathbeds,"

Newsweek, March 24, 1986, 63. Roper is quoted in Cohn, "Behind the Hospital Death Statistics."

30. Cohn, "Behind the Hospital Death Statistics."

31. Gerald Zaltman and Ilan Vertinksy, "Health Services Marketing: A Suggested Model," *Journal of Marketing* 35, no. 3 (July 1971): 19–27.

32. For an insightful account of these developments written in the mid-1980s, see Paul Starr, *The Social Transformation of American Medicine* (New York: Basic Books, 1984), 420–449.

33. Robert Kimmel, "How to Be Ethical While Eating Your Competitor's Lunch," *Marketing Performance: Profiling Tomorrow's Survivors*, Ninth Annual Symposium for Health Care Marketing (Chicago: Academy of Health Care Marketing, American Marketing Association, 1989), 15–16, quotes on 15.

34. Ibid., 16.

35. On the use of advertising to change traditional patterns of physician referral, see, for example, Randall Rothenberg, "Marketing By Hospital is a Success," *New York Times,* December 7, 1988, D17, and "Healthcare Ad Agencies: Prescription for Profit; Growing Competition is Forcing a Major Boost in Medical Marketing Biz," *Adweek*, January 25, 1988.

36. Bruce Allen and Brenda Roberts, "Data Driven Quality Differentiation: Using PRO Mortality Data to Market Your Hospital," in *Marketing Is Everybody's Business*, ed. Peter Sanchez, Eighth Annual Symposium for Health Care Marketing (Chicago: Academy of Health Care Marketing, American Marketing Association., 1988), 165–170, quote on 170.

37. Steven Findlay, Marjory Roberts, and Joanne Silberner, "The Best Hospitals, from AIDS to Urology," *U.S. News and World Report*, April 30, 1990, 68.

38. Ibid.

39. Ibid.; Steven Findlay, "Medicine by the Book," *U.S. News and World Report*, July 6, 1992, 68.

40. Doug Podolsky, "America's Best Hospitals," *U.S. News and World Report*, August 5, 1991, 36. For examples of how local news outlets covered the *U.S. News*'s rankings, see "Local Hospitals among U.S. Best," *Daily News*, July 11, 1999, 13 and "HUP Ranked 10th-Best Hospital in Nation by Magazine Survey," *Philadelphia Inquirer,* July 10, 2000, 1–4.

41. "Who Decides? Frequently Asked Questions about How the Best Doctors Are Chosen," *New York Magazine*, June 18, 2007; Alex Kuckznyski, "Rating of Doctors Now a Business Unto Itself," *New York Times*, March 25, 1999. Bowden quoted in Mark Jurkowitz, "City Mags Bare It, and Grin," *Boston Globe*, June 10, 1999, E1.

42. Margot Heffernan, "The Health Care Quality Improvement Act of 1986 and the National Practitioner Data Bank," *Bulletin of the Medical Library Association* 84, no. 2 (April 1996): 263–269.

43. Ibid., 267. On Public Citizen's dissemination of its own "questionable doctors'" listing, see "Consumer Group is Naming Punished Medical Professionals," *New York Times*, June 29, 1990, A16, and Stuart Auerbach, "Consumer Groups Lists 'Questionable Doctors,'" *Washington Post*, April 9, 1996, Z07.

44. For overviews of these developments, see Preston G. Ribnick and Valerie A. Carrano, "Understanding the New Era in Health Care Accountability: Report Cards," *Journal of Nursing Care Quality* 10 (1995): 1–8; and Millenson, *Demanding Medical Excellence.*

45. "WellPoint Patients Can Give Critiques," *Los Angeles Times*, January 12, 2008.

46. Jean DerGurahian, "Comparative Satisfaction," *Modern Healthcare* 38, no. 13 (March 31, 2008): 6–7. See also "Smart Data, Foolish Choices: Consumers Spurn New Sources of Health Quality Information," *Washington Post*, December 19, 2000; Sandra G. Boodman, "Report Cards for Hospitals," *Washington Post*, December 6, 1994.

47. "Readers Sound off: Best Doctors," *New York Magazine*, July 10, 2006.

48. Judith Hibbard, Jean Stockard, and Martin Tusler, "Hospital Performance Reports: Impact on Quality, Market Share and Reputation," *Health Affairs (Millwood)* 24, no. 4 (2005): 1150–1160.

49. Wendy N. Espeland and Michael Sauder, "Rankings and Reactivity," especially 29–33.

50. Craig R. Narins, Ann M. Dozier, Frederick S. Ling, and Wojciech Zareba, "The Influence of Public Reporting of Outcome Data on Medical Decision Making by Physicians," *Archives of Internal Medicine* 165, no. 1 (January 10, 2005): 83–87; Rachel M. Werner and David A. Asch, "The Unintended Consequences of Publicly Reporting Quality Information," *Journal of the American Medical Association* 293, no. 10 (March 9, 2005): 1239–1244; quote on 1239. See also Robert Kolker, "The Dark Side of Report Cards," *Medical Economics*, 82, no. 23 (December 2, 2005), 69–73.

51. Consumer and Patient Health Information Section, Medical Library Association, "Top 100 List: Health Websites You Can Trust," Medical Library Association Web site, http://caphis.mlanet.org/consumer/ (accessed May 25, 2008).

52. Sanjay Gupta, "Rating Your Doctor," *Time* magazine, January 14, 2008, 62.

53. Epstein, "Cures for an Ailing System."

Chapter 4. When Old Is New

1. Sara Rosenbaum, Phyllis C. Borzi, Lee Repasch, Taylor Burke, John F. Benevelli, *Charting the Legal Environment of Health Information* (George Washington University School of Public Health and Health Services, 2005).

2. HITECH, 42 U.S.C. §13001 et seq. added by Title XVIII, Division A, Pub. I. 111–5, *The American Recovery and Reinvestment Act of 2009*.

3. Catherine DesRoches, Eric G. Campbell, S. R. Rao, K. Donelan, and Timothy G. Ferris et al., "Electronic Health Record Adoption in Ambulatory Settings: A National Survey of Physicians," *New England Journal of Medicine* 359, no. 1 (July 3, 2008): 50–60.

4. Sara Rosenbaum, "The Impact of U.S. Law on Medicine as a Profession," *Journal of the American Medical Association* 289, no. 15 (March 2003): 1546–1556.

5. Timothy Stoltzfus Jost, "The Supreme Court Limits Lawsuits Against Managed Care Organizations," *Health Affairs Web Exclusive* (11 August 2004), w417–w426. http://content.healthaffairs.org/cgi/search?ck=nck&andorexactfulltext=and&resource type=1&disp_type=&author1=&fulltext=Davila&pubdate_year=&volume=& firstpage= (accessed October 20, 2007).

6. Rand E. Rosenblatt, Sylvia A. Law, and Sara Rosenbaum, *Law and the American Health Care System* (New York: Foundation Press, 1997), 28–40.

7. Michelle Mello and David M. Studdert, "The Medical Malpractice System: Structure and Performance," in *Medical Malpractice and the U.S. Health Care System*, ed. William M. Sage and Rogan Kersh (New York: Cambridge University Press, 2006), 11–29; quote on 12.

8. Troyan A. Brennan, Michelle M. Mello, and David M. Studdert, "Liability, Patient Safety, and Defensive Medicine: What Does the Future Hold?" in Sage and Kersh, eds., *Medical Malpractice and the U.S. Health Care System*, 93–114.

9. Rosenblatt, Law, and Rosenbaum, *Law and the American Health Care System*, 843.

10. Ibid., 829–830.

11. See, for example, *Washington v. Washington Hospital Center*, 579 A. 2d 177 (D.C. Ct. App., 1990).

12. David Blumenthal and John P. Glaser, "Information Technology Comes to Medicine," *New England Journal of Medicine* 356, no. 24 (June 14, 2007): 2527.

13. Ibid.

14. 42 C.F.R. §411.351 (2007).

15. Blumenthal and Glaser, "Information Technology Comes to Medicine," 2528.

16. 45 C.F.R. § 164.524; See "Your Health Information Privacy Rights" (United States Department of Health and Human Services) http://www.hhs.gov/ocr/hipaa/consumer _rights.pdf (accessed October 20, 2007).

17. Blumenthal and Glaser, "Information Technology Comes to Medicine," 2528.

18. Ibid., 2528–2529.

19. For an analysis of the importance of interoperability, see Jeff Goldsmith, David Blumenthal, and Wes Rishel, "Federal Health Information Policy: A Case of Arrested Development," *Health Affairs (Millwood)* 22, no. 4 (July/August 2003): 44–55.

20. The controversy over interoperability as a fundamental concept in HIT can be seen in recent federal regulations that condition the granting of legal "safe harbors" against federal fraud prosecution in the case of donated HIT on its interoperability. Legislation introduced during the 109th Congress, when the federal safe harbor regulations were pending, would have clarified that the use of interoperable systems was a voluntary matter. H.R. 4157 §103 (109th Cong. 1st sess.).

21. Jeffrey A. Linder, David W. Bates, Blackford Middleton, and Randall Stafford, "Electronic Health Record Use and the Quality of Ambulatory Care in the U.S.," *Archives of Internal Medicine* 167, no. 13 (July 9, 2004): 1400–1404.

22. Blumenthal and Glaser, "Information Technology Comes to Medicine," 2531.

23. Ibid.

24. Ibid.

25. HHS News Release, "President Directs Federal Agencies to Provide Health Care Quality and Price Information for Consumers," August 22, 2006.

26. *Consumers' Checkbook, Center for Study of Services v. U.S. Dept. of Health and Human Services*, 502 F.Supp.2d 79 (D.D.C., 2007).

27. FTC, *In re Greater Rochester IPA, Advisory Opinion*, Sept. 17, 2007 http://www.ftc.gov/bc/adops/gripa.pdf 14–15 (accessed October 20, 2007).

28. DesRoches et al., "Electronic Health Record Adoption in Ambulatory Settings," 55–57.

29. Charles Bosk, *Forgive and Remember: Managing Medical Failure* (Chicago: University of Chicago Press, 1979); Atul Gawande, *Complications: A Surgeon's Notes on an Imperfect Science* (New York: Henry Holt, 2003).

30. Kristen Madison, "ERISA and Liability for Provision of Medical Information," *North Carolina Law Review* 84 (2006): 471–546, 490.

31. Rosenblatt, Law, and Rosenbaum, *Law and the American Health Care System*, 829–842.

32. Ibid.

33. Mello and Studdert, "Medical Malpractice System: Structure and Performance," 12–13.

34. *Hall v. Hillbun* 466 So. 2d 1985 (Miss., 1985).

35. See the broad review of the learned intermediary doctrine as applied to physicians in Steven R. Kaufman and Jason D. Johnson, "The Learned Intermediary Doctrine and Pharmaceutical Company Liability," *Illinois Bar Journal* 95 (April 2007): 202–212; Lloyd C. Chatfield II, "Medical Implant Litigation and Failure to Warn: A New Extension for the Learned Intermediary Rule?" *Kentucky Law Journal* 82 (Winter 1993/1994): 575–623.

36. Edward Casmere, "Rx for Liability: Advocating the Elimination of the Pharmacist's No Duty to Warn Rule," *John Marshall Law Review* 33 (Winter 2000): 425–453.

37. Cherie N. Wyatt, "Driving on the Center Line: Missouri Physicians' Potential Liability to Third Persons for Failing to Warn of Medication Side Effects," *St. Louis University Law Journal* 46 (2002): 873.

38. Susan A. Casey, "Laying an Old Doctrine to Rest: Challenging the Wisdom of the Learned Intermediary Doctrine," *William Mitchell Law Review* 14 (1993): 931.

39. Tammy R. Wavle, "HIV and AIDS Test Results and the Duty to Warn Third Parties: A Proposal for Uniform Guidelines for Texas Professionals," *St. Mary's Law Journal* 28 (1997): 783.

40. Jeffrey Burnett, "A Physician's Duty to Warn a Patient's Relatives of a Patient's Genetically Inheritable Disease," *Houston Law Review* 36 (1999): 559–609; Sonia M. Suter, "Whose Genes Are These, Anyway? Familial Conflicts over Access to Genetic Information," *Michigan Law Review* 91 (1993): 1854, 1877) (stating that most jurisdictions today would find a duty to warn where a physician has a special relationship with an HIV-infected person, if the victim is both foreseeable and identifiable).

41. Wavle, "HIV and AIDS Test Results and the Duty to Warn Third Parties," 792.

42. Jeffrey J. Wiseman, "Another Factor in the 'Decisional Calculus': The Learned Intermediary Doctrine, the Physician Patient Relationship, and Direct to Consumer Marketing," *South Carolina Law Review* 52 (Summer 2001): 193–216.

43. Peter D. Jacobson and Michael R. Tunick, "Consumer-Directed Health Care and the Courts: Let the Buyer (and Seller) Beware," *Health Affairs (Millwood)* 26, no. 3 (May/June 2007): 704–714.

44. June M. Sullivan, "Physicians as Gatekeepers for Society: Confidentiality of Protected Health Information versus Duty to Disclose At-Risk Drivers," *Health Lawyer* (November 2003): 1–9.

45. Maryann Bobinski, "Autonomy and Privacy: Protecting Patients from Their Physicians," *University of Pittsburgh Law Review* 55 (Winter 1994): 291–360.

46. *Moore v Regents of University of California* 51 Ca1.3d 120 (1990).

47. Bobinski, "Autonomy and Privacy," 306–308.

48. *Canterbury v Spence* 464 F. 2d 272 (USCA DC 1972).

49. Ibid.

50. See cross-jurisdictional discussion of duty of informed consent among diagnosis and treatment alternatives in 38 *American Law Rep.* 900, http://web2.westlaw.com/find/default.wl?rs=WLW7.06&serialnum=1985025930&fn=_top&sv=Split&tc=-1&findtype=Y&tf=-1&db=0000849&utid=%7b6D7129EB-1C8A-420B-AFDF-0025 1A5FFFDE%7d&vr=? 0&rp=%2ffind%2fdefault.wl&mt=LawSchool&RLT=CLID_FQRLT4421177&TF=756&TC=1&n=1 (accessed July 7, 2007).

51. Peter D. Jacobson, "Medical Liability and the Culture of Technology," in Sage and Kersh, eds., *Medical Malpractice and the U.S. Health Care System*, 112–128.

52. 60 F. 2d 737, 739 (2d Cir., 1932).

53. Ibid.

54. 83 Wash. 2d 514 (S. Ct. Wash. State, 1974).

55. 579 A. 2d 177 (D.C. Ct. App., 1990).

56. Jacobson, "Medical Liability and the Culture of Technology," 117.

57. George Annas, "The Patient's Right to Safety—Improving the Quality of Care Through Litigation against Hospitals," *New England Journal of Medicine* 354, no.19 (May 11, 2006): 2063–2066.

58. Ibid.

59. 33 I11.2d 326, 211 N.E.2d 253 (Ill., 1965).

60. Blumenthal and Glaser, "Information Technology Comes to Medicine," 2530; Marlynn Wei, "Doctors, Apologies, and the Law: An Analysis and Critique of Apology Laws," *Journal of Health Law* 40, no. 1 (Winter, 2007): 107–59; *http://www.law.umaryland.edu/academics/journals/jhclp/* (accessed April 17, 2008).

61. Jill Horwitz and Troyan A. Brennan, "No-Fault Compensation for Medical Injury: A Case Study," *Health Affairs (Millwood)* 14, no. 4 (Winter 1995): 165–179.

62. Elizabeth A. McGlynn, S. M. Asch, J. Adams, J. Keesey, J. Hicks, et al., "The Quality of Health Care Delivered to Adults in the United States," *New England Journal of Medicine* 348, no. 26 (June 26, 2003): 2635–2645.

Chapter 5. Patient Data

Acknowledgments: I received helpful comments from Thomas Rice, Lori Andrews, Joel Weissman, Mark Hall, Eugene Declercq, Kristin Madison, and my book co-authors.

1. Marc A. Rodwin, "The Case for Public Ownership of Patient Data," *Journal of the American Medical Association* 302, no. 1 (2009): 86–88; Marc A. Rodwin, "Patient Data: Property, Privacy, and the Public Interest," *American Journal of Law and Medicine* 36, no. 4 (2010) (in press).

2. The market for secondary uses of patient data has its origins in the pharmaceutical industry but is expanding rapidly.

3. Steve Bailey, "Your Data for Sale," *Boston Globe*, March 24, 2006, C1.

4. See Adele A. Waller and Oscar L. Alcantara, "Ownership of Health Information in the Information Age," *Journal of AHIMA* 69, no. 3 (1998): 28–38. However, a better rule is to consider providers as custodians of the medical record. See George J. Annas, *The Rights of Patients: The Authoritative ACLU Guide to the Rights of Patients* (Carbondale: Southern Illinois University Press, 2004), 224–245.

5. Edmund F. Haislmaier, "Health Care Information Technology: Getting the Policy Right," Web Memo No. 1131, (June 16, 2006) (Heritage Foundation), http://www .heritage.org/Research/HealthCare/upload/wm_1131.pdf.

6. "Of the Duties of Physicians to Each Other and the Profession at Large, Art. 1 Duties for the Support of Professional Character, Section 4, American Medical Association, Code of Ethics-1847," in *Ethics in Medicine: Historical Perspectives and Contemporary Concerns* ed. Stanley J. Reiser, Arthur J. Dyck, and William J. Curran (Cambridge, MA: MIT Press, 1977), 26–34.

7. *AMA Principles of Medical Ethics*, 2001, V. "A physician shall continue to study, apply, and advance scientific knowledge, maintain a commitment to medical education, make relevant information available to patients, colleagues, and the public, obtain consultation, and use the talents of other health professionals when indicated." *AMA Principles of Medical Ethics*, 1980, V. "A physician shall continue to study, apply and advance scientific knowledge, make relevant information available to patients, colleagues, and the public, obtain consultation, and use the talents of other health professionals when indicated." *AMA Principles of Medical Ethics*, 1957, Section 2. "Physicians should strive continually to improve medical knowledge and

skill, and should make available to their patients and colleagues the benefits of their professional attainments." Reiser, Dyck, and Curran, eds., *Ethics in Medicine*.

8. American Board of Internal Medicine Foundation, American College of Physicians-American Society of Internal Medicine Foundation and European Federation of Internal Medicine, "Medical Professionalism in the New Millennium: A Physician Charter," *Annals of Internal Medicine* 136, no. 3 (2002): 243–246.

9. Ben Gaffin, "Report on a Study of Advertising and the American Physician, Pt. 1," in *Hearing before the Subcommittee on Antitrust and Monopoly of the Committee on the Judiciary*, 505, 1961–1962, reprinted in U.S. Congress, Senate, Hearing before the Subcommittee on Antitrust and Monopoly of the Committee on the Judiciary, "*Drug Industry Antitrust Act (S. 1551)*," 8th Cong., 1st and 2nd session (1961–1962), pt.1, 505.

10. Jeremy A. Green, "Pharmaceutical Marketing Research and the Prescribing Physician," *Annals of Internal Medicine* 146, no. 10 (2007): 742–747.

11. Ibid.

12. Robert Steinbrook, "For Sale: Physicians' Prescribing Data," *New England Journal of Medicine* 354, no. 26 (2006): 2745–2747.

13. Data obtained from the AMA identified physicians by their practice specialty, affiliations with hospitals and insurers, practice location, and other variables. Information from pharmacies and other firms revealed information on drugs prescribed and sold. Combining such information reveals individual physician and aggregate prescribing patterns. Similar information allows firms to track the use of medical devices and other medical products. Electronic medical records expand the kind and volume of patient data available. They reveal the profile of patients treated by individual physicians and hospitals and the particular diagnosis of patients for whom drugs and medical devices are prescribed.

14. Joe Priest, "Hospital-Centric Prescription Data Opens New Patient Level Insights and Marketing Opportunities," *Pharmaceutical Commerce* (August 20, 2007), http://www.pharmaceuticalcommerce.com/frontEnd/main.php?idSeccion=677; Jean-Patrick Tsang, "Patient-Data Comes of Age," *Pharmaceutical Executive* (May 1, 2003), http://pharmexec.findpharma.com/pharmexec/PE+Features/Patient-Data-Come-of-Age/ArticleLong/Article/detail/55300.

15. Taryi Forni, "Using Patient-Level Data to Take Your Market Assessment to the Next Level," *Journal of Longitudinal Data* (January/February 2005): 12–17; Forni, "Using Anonymous Patient-Level Information to Inform the Brand-Planning Process: Part 2," *Product Management Today* (May 2006): 14–15; Julie Klossner and Jack Newson, "Studying Drug Utilization by Production Indication," *Product Management Today* (October 2005): 16–17; Taryi Forni and Zohar Porat, "Assessing Treatment Patterns in Complex Disease Markets: An Example from the Mental Health Market," *Product Management Today* (April 2005): 12–13; John Martin and Stephen J. Boccuzzi, "Analyzing Drug Utilization Patterns in the Oncology Market," *Product Management Today* (March 2006): 14–15.

10. IMS, "Annual Report 2007 10-K Sec Registration Statement," 2007.

17. IMS, "Health Economics and Outcomes Research, Generating Creative and Informative Content for the Pharmaceutical, Science and Medical Fields," http://www.imshealth.com/web/channel/0,3147,64576068_63872702_73163984,00.html.

18. IMS, "Health Economics and Outcomes Research, Medical Writing and Communication," http://www.imshealth.com/web/channel/0,3147,77141581_63872702_77140611,00.html.

19. Ibid.

20. See American Health Information Management Association, August 3, Letter of Jonathan White in Response to National Health Data Stewardship Entity, www.ahima.org/dc/documents/MicrosoftWord-AHIMANHDSERFIresponse -final_2007–08–03.pdf (accessed January 6, 2010).

21. IMS, "Annual Report 2007 10-K SEC Registration Statement," 3.

22. IMS, "Annual Report 2007 10-K SEC Registration Statement," 7.

23. "National Health Data Stewardship," *Federal Register* 72, no. 106 (2007): 30803–30805.

24. See American Health Information Management Association, "Development of a National Health Data Stewardship Entity."

25. "Connecting for Health, July 30, 2007, Letter from P. John White in response to request for information regarding a National Data Stewardship Entity. Available at http://www.connectingforhealth.org/resources/cth_ahrq_aqa_rfi_073007.pdf (accessed January 6, 2010).

26. The National Commission on Quality Assurance; The National Quality Forum; The Joint Commission. Response to National Health Data Stewardship Request for Information (FR Doc. 07–2733): Submitted to AHRQ Department of Health and Human Services, July 27, 2007, http://healthit.ahrq.gov/portal/server.pt? CommunityID=666&PageID=0&Submit.x=1&Submit.y=1&control=SetCommunity& in_tx_query=ncqa&space=CommunityPage&spaceID=399 (accessed June 1, 2009).

27. Ibid., 15.

28. David M. Eddy, "Evidence-Based Medicine: A Unified Approach," *Health Affairs (Millwood)* 24, no. 1 (2005): 9–17.

29. Jonathan B. Perlin and Joel Kupersmith, "Information Technology and the Inferential Gap," *Health Affairs (Millwood)* 26, no. 2 (2007): w192–w194.

30. Lynn M. Etheredge, "A Rapid-Learning Health System," *Health Affairs (Millwood)* 26, no. 2 (2007): w107–w118. Walter F. Stewart, Nirav R. Shah, Mark J. Selna, Ronald A. Paulus, and James M. Walker, "Bridging the Inferential Gap: The Electronic Health Record and Clinical Evidence," *Health Affairs (Millwood)* 26, no. 2 (2007): w181–w191.

31. One research team purchased such prescription data from IMS to identify such practices. See David C. Radley, Stan N. Finkelstein, and Randall S. Stafford, "Off-Label Prescribing among Office-Based Physicians," *Archives of Internal Medicine* 166, no. 9 (2006): 1021–1026; David W. Bates, Benjamin Honigman, Joshua Lee, Jeffrey Rothschild, Patrice Light, Russell M. Pulling, and Tony Yu, "Using Computerized Data to Identify Adverse Drug Events in Outpatients," *Journal of the American Medical Informatics Association* 8 (2001): 254–266.

32. Some of the limitations of observational data from patient records can be addressed when the data is used in simulation models. See John R. Lumpkin, "Archimedes: A Bold Step into the Future," *Health Affairs (Millwood)* 26, no. 2 (2007): w137–w139; David M. Eddy, "Linking Electronic Medical Records to Large-Scale Simulation Models: Can We Put Rapid Learning on Turbo?" *Health Affairs (Millwood)* 26, no. 2 (2007): w125–w136; R. I. Horowitz et al., "Developing Improved Observational Methods for Evaluating Therapeutic Effectiveness," *American Journal of Medicine* 89, no. 5 (1990): 630–638.

33. RTI International, "Recommended Requirements for Enhancing Data Quality in Electronic Health Record Systems," 4–6. Washington, D.C.: Office of the National Coordinator for Health Information Technology, Department of Health and Human

Services, 2007. http://www.rti.org/pubs/enhancing_data_quality_in_ehrs.pdf. American Health Management Association, "Development of a National Health Data Stewardship Entity" at p. 12.

34. Etheredge, "Rapid-Learning Health System." w107–w118.

35. Joel Kupersmith, Joseph Francis, Eve Kerr, Sarah Krein, Leonard Pogach, Robert M. Kolodner, and Jonathan B. Perlin, "Advancing Evidence-Based Care for Diabetes: Lessons From the Veteran's Health Administration," *Health Affairs (Millwood)* 6, no. 2 (2007): w156–w168.

36. Stewart et al., "Bridging the Inferential Gap," w181–w191.

37. CMS, "Medicare Prescription Drug Data Strategy: Improving Evidence for Patient Care through the Medicare Prescription Drug Benefit," http://www.medicarerxguide .com/MDRG/2005/CMS_Data_Strategy_for_Part_D.pdf.

38. Sean R. Tunis, Tanisha V. Carino, Reginald D. Williams II, and Peter B. Bach, "Federal Initiative to Support Rapid Learning About New Technologies," *Health Affairs (Millwood)* 26, no. 2 (2007): w140–w149.

39. CDC/ATSDR, "Policy on Releasing and Sharing Data Manual Guide: General Administration, CDC-102," http://www.cdc.gov/od/foia/policies/sharing.htm.

40. The reporting began with the passage of the California Hospital Disclosure Act by the California Legislature, Senate Bill 283, in 1971. Since then the reporting requirements have been revised through legislation and regulation several times. For a history, see http://www.oshpd.ca.gov/mircal/programs/IP/patmanuals/pd3/Part%202 %20-%20INTRODUCTION.pdf. For information on the availability of the data and a manual that describes the data, see Office of Statewide Health Planning and Development, "Medical Information Reporting for California (Mircal)," http://www .oshpd.ca.gov/mircal/programs/IP/PDSManual.htm.

41. G. Dietlin and D. Schroder-Bernhardi, "Use of the Mediplus Patient Database in Healthcare Research," *International Journal of Clinical Pharmacology and Therapeutics* 40, no. 3 (2002): 130–133.

42. Letter from W. David Helms, Ph.D., on behalf of Academy Health to Agency for Healthcare Research and Quality in response to *Federal Register* request for comments, July 26, 2007, http://www.chsr.org/AHRQRFI (accessed June 2, 2009).

43. Charles Safran, Merly Bloomrosen, and W. Edward Hammond, "Toward a National Framework for the Secondary Use of Health Data: An American Medical Informatics Association White Paper," *Journal of American Medical Informatics Association* 14, no. 1 (2007): 1–9.

44. Ibid., 3.

45. Ibid., 6.

46. Ibid., 6. The AMIA reasserted that view recently. See, American Health Management Association, "Development of a National Health Data Stewardship Entity," at p. 4.

47. The AMIA provides model contracts to members to protect information as proprietary.

48. See Jill Burrington-Brown, Beth Hjort, and Lydia Washington, "Health Data Access, Use, and Control," *Journal of AHIMA* 78, no. 5 (2007): 63–66; Burrington-Brown, Hjort, and Washington, "Health Data Access, Use and Control," http://library .ahima.org/xpedio/groups/public/documents/ahima/bok1_034053.hcsp?dDocName= bok1_034053.

49. The Department of Health and Human Services requested comments on a National Health Data Stewardship Entity in the summer of 2007. See Department of Health and Human Services, "Agency for Healthcare Research and Quality: National Health

Data Stewardship," *Federal Register* 72, no. 106 (June 4, 2007): 30803–30805. The idea was harshly criticized by industry in its comments to DHHS.

50. Bailey, "Your Data for Sale."

51. The TRIPS Agreement is Annex 1C of the *Marrakesh Agreement Establishing the World Trade Organization*, signed in Marrakesh, Morocco, on April 15, 1994. Article 39.3 of TRIPS applies to clinical trial test data. Carlos M. Correa, "Protecting Test Data from Pharmaceutical and Agrochemical Products under Free Trade Agreements," in *Negotiating Health: Intellectual Property and Access to Medicine*, ed. Pedro Roffe, Geoff Tansey, and David Vivas Eugui (London: Earthscan, 2006), 81–97; Mier Perez Pugtach, "Intellectual Property, Data Exclusivity, Innovation and Market Access," in Roffe, Tansey, and Eugui, eds., *Negotiating Health,,* 97–132. Robert Weisman, "Data Protection: Options for Implementation," in Roffe, Tansey, and Eugui, eds., *Negotiating Health,* 151–180.

52. Jerome H. Reichman, "The International Legal Status of Undisclosed Clinical Trial Data: From Private to Public Goods?" in Roffe, Tansey, and Eugui, eds., *Negotiating Health,* 133–150.

53. Gregory D. Curfman, Stephen Morrissey, and Jeffrey M. Drazen, "Expression of Concern: Bombardier et al. "Comparison of Upper Gastrointestinal Toxicity of Rofecoxib and Naproxen in Patients with Rheumatoid Arthritis," *New England Journal of Medicine* 343 (2000): 1520–1528," *New England Journal of Medicine* 353, no. 26 (December 29, 2000): 2813–2814. See John Abramson, "False and Misleading: The Misrepresentation of Celebrex and Vioxx," in his book, *Overdo$ed America: The Broken Promise of American Medicine* (New York: HarperCollins, 2004), 23–38.

54. Catherine D. De Angelis, Jeffrey M. Drazen, Frank A. Frizelle et al., "Clinical Trial Registration: A Statement from the International Committee of Medical Journal Editors," *New England Journal of Medicine* 351, no. 12 (2004): 1250–1251. Christine R. Laine, Richard Horton, Catherine. D. De Angelis et al., "Clinical Trial Registration—Looking Back and Moving Ahead," *New England Journal of Medicine* 356, no. 26 (2007): 2734–2736.

55. Jeffrey M. Drazen, Stephen Morrissey, and Gregory D. Curfman, "Open Clinical Trials," *New England Journal of Medicine* 357, no. 17 (2007): 1756–1757.

56. Copyright Act of 1976, Public Law Number 94–553, *Food and Drug Administration Revitalization Act,* Public Law 110–80.

57. *Feist Publications v. Rural Telephone Service Co,* 499 U.S. 360 (1991).

58. In 1996, the European Union (EU) adopted a directive that protects the content of databases when they are original due to selection or arrangement of their contents. The directive extends this protection to nationals of other countries where the other country offers comparable protection to EU databases. (EPC, "Directive 96/9/Ec of the European Parliament and of the Council of 11 March 1996," in *Directive on the Legal Protection of Databases,* 20–28, 1996). Also in 1996, legislation was introduced in the U.S. Congress to grant special protection for databases. The U.S. Copyright Office has studied the pros and cons of granting new legal protection for databases and analyzed the principles and interests at stake. It notes competing considerations. For example, it says that copyright should not harm science, research, education, or reporting but it also says that "substantial copying for commercial, competitive purposes should not be permitted." See H.R. 35231, Database Investment and Intellectual Property Anti-Piracy Act of 1996. Database and Collections of Information Misappropriation Act of 2003.Those bills were not enacted, nor were

similar bills introduced in 2003. "U.S. Copyright Office Report on Legal Protections for Databases." U.S. Copyright Office, http://www.copyright.gov/reports/dbase.html. The Subcommittee on Courts, the Internet, and Intellectual Property, Committee on the Judiciary and the Subcommittee on Commerce, Trade and Consumer Protection Committee on Energy and Commerce, *Statement of David O. Carson, General Counsel, United States Copyright Office*, September 23, 2003, http://www.copyright .gov/docs/regstat092303.html. Copyright Office for Senator Orrin Hatch, "Executive Summary, U.S. Copyright Office Report on Legal Protections for Databases, ix," edited by U.S. Copyright Office. http://www.copyright.gov/reports/exsum.pdf.

59. Waller, "Ownership of Health Information," 33.

60. Ibid., 32.

61. Richard A. Musgrave, "A Multiple Theory of Budget Determination," *FinanzArchiv* 25, no. 1 (1957): 33–43. Musgrave, "Merit Goods," in *The New Palgrave Dictionary of Economics*, ed. Steven N. Durlauf and Lawrence E. Blume, 2nd ed. (Hampshire, England: Palgrave Macmillan, 2008), vol. 5.

62. There is probably also some value to organizations generating additional data that might also yield spillover benefits. There is thus a case for treating such new data as a merit good and for the government subsidizing its production.

63. As a legal matter, property consists of a bundle of rights, which can be divided in numerous ways. It is possible for one person to possess all these rights. However, it is also possible for various parties to have different property rights in one entity. For example, ownership of land can be divided so that one person has grazing rights, another rights to extract minerals, a third rights to use underground water, a fourth to construct a building on the land, and a fifth to have a right of way to cross the land. These rights may also be limited to different time periods and subject to various restrictions or conditions.

64. The phrase "the tragedy of the commons" was coined by Garrett Hardin in his classic essay, "The Tragedy of the Commons," *Science* 162, no. 3859 (1968): 1243–1248.

65. Many writers emphasize the value of private ownership to avoid the tragedy of the commons. But management of the publicly owned resource can be equally effective. The later possibility is often forgotten but discussed in the thoughtful literature on this subject and by Garrett Hardin in his review of the issues thirty years after his first essay. See, Garrett Hardin, "Extensions of 'The Tragedy of the Commons,'" *Science* 280, no. 5364 (1998): 682–683.

66. Michael A. Heller and Rebecca Eisenberg, "Can Patents Deter Innovation? The Anticommons in Biomedical Research," *Science* 280, no. 5364 (1998): 698–701; quote on 698; Michael A. Heller, "The Tragedy of the Anticommons: Property in the Transition from Marx to Markets," *Harvard Law Review* 111, no. 3 (1998): 621–688; Scott Stern and Fiona E Murray, "Do Formal Intellectual Property Rights Hinder the Free Flow of Scientific Knowledge? An Empirical Test of the Anti-Commons Hypothesis," in *NBER Working Paper No. W11465*, Available at SSRN: 2005, http://papers.ssrn.com/s013/papers.cfm?abstract_id=755701; James M. Buchanan and Yong J. Yoon, "Symmetric Tragedies: Commons and Anticommons," *Journal of Law and Economics* 43, no. 1 (2000): 1–14; Margaret Jane Radin, "Property Evolving in Cyberspace," *Journal of Law and Commerce* 15, no. 2 (1996): 509–525; Hanoch Dagan and Michael A. Heller, "The Liberal Commons," *Yale Law Journal* 110, no. 4 (2001): 549–623.

67. Carl Shapiro, "Navigating the Patent Thicket: Cross Licenses, Patent Pools, and Standard-Setting," in *Innovation Policy and the Economy*, ed. Adam B. Jaffe, Josh

Lerner, and Scott Stern (Cambridge, MA: MIT Press, 2001), vol. 1, 119–150. http://www.nber.org/confer/2000/ipes00/shapiro.pdf.

68. These examples and the discussion are based on Lori B. Andrews, "Genes and Patent Policy: Rethinking Intellectual Property Rights," *Nature Reviews: Genetics* 3, no. 10 (2002): 803–808. The analysis of these problems is developed further in Lori B. Andrews and Jordan Paradise, "Gene Patents: The Need for Bioethics Scrutiny and Legal Change," *Yale Journal of Health Policy, Law & Ethics*. 5, no. 1 (2005): 403–412; Jordan Paradise, Lori B. Andrews, and Timothy Holbrook, "Intellectual Property: Patents on Human Genes: An Analysis of Scope and Claims," *Science* 307, no. 5715 (2005): 1566–1567.

69. U.S. Patent No. 5,508,167.

70. E.U. Patent No. EP699754.

71. Harlan J. Onsrud, "The Tragedy of the Information Commons," in *Policy Issues in Modern Cartography*, ed. D. R. F. Taylor (Oxford: Elsevier Science, 1998), 141–158.

72. Pamela Samuelson, "Privacy as Intellectual Property," *Stanford Law Review* 52, no. 5 (2000): 1125–1174; Vera Bergelson, "It's Personal but It's Mine? Toward Property Rights in Personal Information," *U.C. Davis Law Review* 37, no. 2 (2003): 379–451; Daniel D. Branhizer, "Symposium: Cyber persons, Propertization, and Contract in the Information Culture: Propitiation Metaphors for Bargaining Power and Control of the Self in the Information Age," *Cleveland State Law Review* 54, no. 1, pt. 2 (2006): 69–113; Sonia M. Suter, "Disentangling Privacy from Property: Toward a Deeper Understanding of Genetic Privacy," *George Washington Law Review* 72, no. 4 (2004): 737–814. For a sample of those opposed to making personal information property, see Anita L. Allen, "Coercing Privacy," *William and Mary Law Review* 40, no. 3 (1999): 723–757; Julie E. Cohen, "Examined Lives: Informational Privacy and the Subject as Object," *Stanford Law Review* 52, no. 5 (2000): 1373–1438; Mark A. Lemley, "Private Property," *Stanford Law Review* 52, no. 5 (2000): 1545–1557; and Marc Rotenberg, "Fair Information Practices and the Architecture of Privacy," *Stanford Technology Law Review* 1 (2001): 92–97.

73. See, *AMA Principles of Medical Ethics*, 2001. IV. "A physician shall respect the rights of patients, colleagues, and other health professionals, and shall safeguard patient confidences and privacy within the constraints of the law." *AMA Principles of Medical Ethics*, 1980, IV. "A physician shall respect the rights of patients, colleagues, and of other health professionals, and shall safeguard patient confidences within the constraints of the law." *AMA Principles of Medical Ethics*, 1957, "Section 9. A physician may not reveal the confidences entrusted to him in the course of medical attendance, or the deficiencies he may observe in the character of patients, unless he is required to do so by law or unless it becomes necessary in order to protect the welfare of the individual or of the community." Reiser, Dyck, and Curran, eds. *Ethics in Medicine*; AMA CEJA Opinion, "5.075 Disclosure of Records to Data Collection Companies."

74. In most states, patients' medical records are available to patients, providers, as well as hospitals and other institutions that provide medical services. Patients have a right to obtain copies of their medical records. They may have their medical records transferred to another physician if they change doctors. Hospitals and other institutions can keep copies of patient medical records after patients are discharged.

75. Even when patient privacy interest is not compromised, patients still have other interests in how information from their medical records is used. They have interests in such information being used to improve medical care for themselves and others.

They may also have interests in sharing the commercial gain from such information or in restricting the use of such information in ways that harm patients or compromise good medical practice. The interest in data resembles, in part, that of research subjects in how their tissue or cells are used. For analysis of the interest of research subjects, see Lori A. Andrews and Julie Burger, "A Pound of Flesh: Patient Legal Action for Human Research Protection in the Biotech Age," in Beatrice Hoffman, Nancy Tomes, Rachel Grob, et al. eds., *Impatient Voices: Patients as Policy Actors* (New Brunswick, NJ: Rutgers University Press, forthcoming 2011).

76. *Tarasoff v. Regents of the University of California*, 17 Cal. 3d 425, 551 P.2d 334, 131 Cal. Rptr. 14 (Cal. 1976).

77. Department of Health and Human Services, 5 Code of Federal Regulations, Parts 160 and 164, "Standards for Privacy of Individually Identifiable Health Data," *Federal Register* 67, no. 157 (August 14, 2002), 53182–53273.

78. 45 Code of Federal Regulation § 164.514(a).

79. Paul Schwartz and Joel R. Reidenberg, "Data Privacy Law: A Study of United States Data Protection" (Charlottesville, VA: Michie, 1996), chapter 5.

80. "Developments in the Law—the Law of Cyberspace," *Harvard Law Review* 112 no. 7 (1999): 1574–1586; Kenneth C. Laudon, "Markets and Privacy," *Communications of the Association of Computing Machinery (ACM)* 39, no. 9 (1996): 92–104; Lawrence Lessig, *Code: And Other Laws of Cyberspace* (New York: Basic Books, 1999); Lawrence Lessig, "The Architecture of Privacy," *Vanderbilt Journal of Entertainment Law & Practice* 1 (1999): 56–65; Patricia Mell, "Seeking Shade in a Land of Perpetual Sunlight: Privacy as Property in the Electronic Wilderness," *Berkeley Technology Journal* 1, no 1 (1996): 26–41; Bergelson, "It's Personal but It's Mine?" 379–451.

81. Laudon, "Markets and Privacy," 92–104. Radin, "Property Evolving in Cyberspace," 516–517.

82. Samuelson. "Privacy as Intellectual Property."

83. See Joseph L. Sax, "Takings, Private Property and Private Rights," *Yale Law Journal* 81, no. 2 (1971): 149–186; *Lucas v. South Carolina Coastal Council*, 505 U.S. 1003 (1992).

84. I am indebted to Eugene Declercq for helping me understand the limitations of data.

85. "Sick Around the World," *Frontline*, April 15, 2005, *http://www.pbs.org/wgbh/pages/frontline/sickaroundtheworld/view/main.html*.

Chapter 6. The Impact of Information Technology on Organ Donation

1. Organ Procurement Transplant Network, "All Kaplan-Meir Graft Survival Rates for Transplants Performed: 1997–2004" (April 25, 2008), http://www.optn.org/latestData/rptStrat.asp (accessed from the OPTN/UNOS Web site on April 30, 2008).

2. Organ Procurement Transplant Network, "Kidney Kaplan-Meier Patient Survival Rates for Transplants Performed: 1997–2004" (April 25, 2008), http://www.optn.org/latestData/rptStrat.asp (accessed from the OPTN/UNOS Web site on April 30, 2008).

3. Organ Procurement Transplant Network, "Overall by Organ Current U.S. Waiting List" (April 25, 2008), http://www.optn.org/latestData/rptData.asp (accessed from the OPTN/UNOS Web site on April 30, 2008). Numbers may be inflated. See Rob Stein, "A Third of Patients on Transplant List Are Not Eligible," *Washington Post*, March 22, 2008.

4. Organ Procurement Transplant Network, "Death Removals by Region by Year" (April 25, 2008), http://www.optn.org/latestData/rptData.asp (accessed from the OPTN/UNOS Web site on April 30, 2008).

5. David J. Rothman, *Strangers at the Bedside: A History of How Law and Bioethics Transformed Medical Decision Making* (New York: Basic Books, 1991).

6. D. Sanders and J. Dukeminier, Jr., "Medical Advance and Legal Lag: Hemodialysis and Kidney Transplantation," *UCLA Law Review* 15 (1968): 357–413; quote on 378.

7. Rothman, *Strangers at the Bedside.*

8. Organ Procurement Transplant Network, "Transplants by Donor Type" (April 25, 2008), http://www.optn.org/latestData/rptData.asp (accessed from the OPTN/UNOS Web site on April 30, 2008).

9. Organ Procurement Transplant Network, "Living Donor Transplants By Donor Relation" (April 25, 2008), http://www.optn.org/latestData/rptData.asp (accessed from the OPTN/UNOS Web site on April 30, 2008).

10. Matchingdonors, "About Matchingdonors.com.," http://matchingdonors.com/life/index.cfm?page=main&frm=about (accessed on April 20, 2008); S. Allen, "Web-Based Kidney Match Raises Ethics Questions," *Boston Globe*, October 20, 2004; Robert D. Truog, "The Ethics of Organ Donation by Living Donors," *New England Journal of Medicine* 353, no. 5 (2005): 444–446; Susan Aschoff, "Out of Line?" *St. Petersburg Times (Florida)*, April 17, 2005.

11. Matchingdonors, www.matchingdonors.com (accessed on April 7, 2008); Rob Stein, "Search for Transplant Organs Becomes a Web Free-for-All," *Washington Post*, September 23, 2005; M. Garvey, "Some Jumping the Line on Organ Transplants; with Waiting Lists and Waiting Times Growing, a Small but Increasing Number of Patients Take Unusual Approaches to Find Matching Donors," *Los Angeles Times*, October 24, 2005; S. Jacobs, "Online Organ Linkups Spur Debate," *Boston Globe*, December 3, 2004; Truog, "Ethics of Organ Donation by Living Donors," 444–446; Aschoff, "Out of Line?"

12. J. Coupland, "Dating Advertisements: Discourses of the Commodified Self," *Discourse and Society* 7 no. 2 (1996): 187–207.

13. M. Hardey, "Mediated Relationships, Authenticity, and the Possibility of Romance," *Information, Communications, and Society* 7, no. 2 (June 2004): 207–222. Coupland, "Dating Advertisements," 187–207. N. Fairclough, "Critical Discourse Analysis and the Marketization of Public Discourse: The Universities," *Discourse and Society* 4, no 2. (1995): 133–168.

14. C. Gillette, "Reputation and Intermediaries in Electronic Commerce," *Louisiana University Law Review* 63 (2002): 1165–1199.

15. Robert D. Putnam, *The Collapse and Revival of American Community* (New York: Simon and Schuster, 2000).

16. Manuel Castells, "The Internet and the Network Society," in *The Internet in Everyday Life*, ed. Barry Wellman and Caroline Haythornthwaite (Oxford and Malden, MA: Blackwell Publishers, 2002), xxix; Manuel Castells, "Materials for an Exploratory Theory of the Network Society," *British Journal of Sociology* 51, no. 1 (January/March 2000): 5–24; Manuel Castells, *The Internet Galaxy: Reflections on the Internet, Business, and Society* (Oxford: Oxford University Press, 2001); Andrew Feenberg and Darin Barney, eds., *Community in the Digital Age: Philosophy and Practice* (New York: Rowman and Littlefield, 2004); Barry Wellman, "Physical Place and Cyberplace: The Rise of Personalized Networking," *International Journal of Urban and Regional Research* 25, no. 2 (2001): 227–252; Barry Wellman and Milena Gulia, "Virtual Communities as Communities: Net Surfers Don't Ride Alone," in *Communities in Cyberspace*, ed. Marc A. Smith and Peter Kollock (London: Routledge, 1999), 167–194.

17. Manuel Castells, "Internet and Network Society," in Wellman, ed., *Internet in Everyday Life*, xxxi; Manuel Castells, *The Rise of the Network Society*, 2nd ed. (Oxford and Malden, MA: Blackwell Publishing, 2000).

18. Lee Rainie, John Horrigan, Barry Wellman, Jeffrey Boase, "The Strength of Internet Ties," Pew Internet and American Life Project, January 25, 2006, 42, http://www.pewinternet.org/Reports/2006/The-Strength-of-Internet-Ties.aspx (accessed January 8, 2010).

19. Ibid.

20. Roberta G. Simmons, *Gift of Life: The Social and Psychological Impact of Organ Donation* (New York: Wiley-Interscience, 1977), 313–314.

21. Ibid., 323.

22. Felicia Wu Song, "Virtual Communities in a Therapeutic Age." *Society*, January/February 2002; George Simmel, "The Stranger," in *George Simmel on Individuality and Social Forms*, ed. Donald N. Levine (Chicago: University of Chicago Press, 1971).

23. Song, "Virtual communities," 44.

24. Ibid, 44.

25. Ibid.

26. R. Epstein, "The Truth about Online Dating," *Scientific American Mind* 20, issue 30 (January 30, 2009), 54–62.

27. Sherry Turkle, "Looking Toward Cyberspace: Beyond Grounded Sociology: Cyberspace and Identity," *Contemporary Sociology* 28, no. 6 (November 1999): 643–648; Sherry Turkle, "Our Split Screens," Etnofoor issue 15 (December 2002), 5–20; Sherry Turkle, *Life on the Screen: Identity in the Age of the Internet* (New York: Simon and Schuster, 1995).

28. William Curran, "A Problem of Consent: Kidney Transplantation in Minors," *NYU Law Review*, 34 (1959): 891–898.

29. National Telecommunications and Information Association, "Falling through the Net: A Survey of the 'Have-Nots' in Rural and Urban America," 1995, http://www.ntia.doc.gov/ntiahome/fallingthru.html(accessed April 28, 2008).

30. Susannah Fox, "Pew Report: Digital Divisions," October 5, 2005, Pew Internet and American Life Project, http://www.pewinternet.org/PPF/r/165/report_display.asp (accessed April 28, 2008).

31. United Network for Organ Sharing (2004), UNOS Board Meeting. Authors of this chapter were present and taking minutes. June 24–25, 2004, Minneapolis, Minnesota.

32. Stein, "Search for Transplant Organs Becomes a Web Free-for-All."

33. R. Metzger, "Memorandum Addresses Living Donor Solicitation," UNOS Memo to the Board of Directors, January 12, 2005. http://www.unos.org/news/newsDetail .asp?id=391 (accessed on the UNOS Web site on January 8, 2010).

34. A. Friedman, "Patient Access to Transplantation: With an Internet-Identified Live Kidney Donor: A Survey of U.S. Centers," *Transplantation* 85, no. 6 (March 27, 2008): 794–798.

35. See American Board of Internal Medicine Foundation, American College of Physicians-American Society of Internal Medicine Foundation, and European Federation of Internal Medicine, "Medical Professionalism in the New Millennium: A Physician Charter," *Annals of Internal Medicine* 136, no. 3 (February 5, 2002): 243.

36. E-mail exchanges between two transplant surgeons on the Centerspan email listserv, December 9, 2009.

37. Truog, "Ethics of Organ Donation by Living Donors," 444–446.

Chapter 7. Changing the Rules

1. Hannah Rion, *The Truth about Twilight Sleep* (New York: McBride & Nast, 1915).
2. Eugene R. Declercq, C. Sakala, M. P. Corry, and S. Applebaum, *Listening to Mothers II: Report of the Second National U.S. Survey of Women's Childbearing Experiences* (New York: Childbirth Connection, 2006).
3. Judy Barrett Litoff, *American Midwives: 1860 to the Present* (Westport, CT: Greenwood Press, 1978).
4. Raymond Devries, Sirpa Wrede, Edwin R. van Teijlingen, and Cecilia Benoit, eds., *Birth by Design: Pregnancy, Maternity Care, and Midwifery in North America and Europe* (New York: Routledge, 2001).
5. Richard W. Wertz and Dorothy C. Wertz, *Lying-in: A History of Childbirth in America* (New York: Schocken Books, 1977).
6. H. S. Williams, *Painless Childbirth* (New York: Goodhue Company, 1914).
7. Wertz and Wertz, *Lying-in*, 150–154.
8. Rion, *Truth about Twilight Sleep.*
9. Barbara Bridgman Perkins, *The Medical Delivery Business: Health Reform, Childbirth, and the Economic Order* (New Brunswick, NJ: Rutgers University Press, 2003).
10. K. DeGeorges, P. Van Hine, and W. Pearse, "ACOGQUEST: The Model Phase of the IAIMS Project of the American College of Obstetricians and Gynecologists," *Bulletin of the Medical Library Association* 80, no. 3 (1992): 276–280; P. Van Hine and W. Pearse, "The IAIMS Project of the American College of Obstetricians and Gynecologists: Using Information Technology to Improve the Health Care of Women," *Bulletin of the Medical Library Association* 76, no. 3 (1988): 237–241.
11. Van Hine and Pearse, "IAIMS Project."
12. Catherine Corey and Joy M. Grossman, *Clinical Information Technology Adoption Varies across Physician Specialties* (Washington, D.C.: Center for Studying Health System Change, 2007), http://www.hschange.org/CONTENT/935/?topic=topic 22.
13. Michael T. Mennuti, "Embracing Change in Obstetrics and Gynecology," *Obstetrics & Gynecology* 106, no. 5, pt. 1 (2005): 905.
14. U.S. House of Representatives, Subcommittee on Health of the House Committee on Ways and Means, Hearing, Testimony of Michael Mennuti, President, American College of Obstetricians and Gynecologists," on *The Medicare Value-Based Purchasing for Physicians Act* (September 29, 2005), 109th Congress, 1st session, Serial 109–42 (2005).
15. Iain Chalmers, Murray Enkin, and Marc J. N. C. Keirse, eds., *Effective Care in Pregnancy and Childbirth* (Oxford: Oxford University Press, 1989).
16. Iain Chalmers, "The Epidemiology of Perinatal Practice," *Journal of Maternal and Child Health* 4 (1979): 435–436.
17. D. A. Grimes, M. Y. Hou, L. M. Lopez, and K. Nanda, "Do Clinical Experts Rely on the Cochrane Library?" [Editorial], *Obstetrics & Gynecology* 111, no. 2, pt 1 (2008): 420–422.
18. Stephen Thacker, D. Stroup, and M. Chang, "Continuous Electronic Heart Rate Monitoring for Fetal Assessment during Labor," *Cochrane Database of Systematic Reviews* 2000; CD000063. DOI: 10.1002/14651858.CD000063.pub2(1), http://www.cochrane.org/reviews/htm/.
19. M. G. Rosen and J. C. Dickinson, "The Paradox of Electronic Fetal Monitoring: More Data May Not Enable Us to Predict or Prevent Infant Neurologic Morbidity," *American Journal of Obstetrics & Gynecology* 168, no. 3, pt. 3 (1993): 745–751.

20. K. B. Nelson, J. M. Dambrosia, T. Y. Ting, and J. K. Grether, "Uncertain Value of Electronic Fetal Monitoring in Predicting Cerebral Palsy," *New England Journal of Medicine* 334, no. 10 (1996): 613–618.

21. J. T. Parer and T. King, "Fetal Heart Rate Monitoring: Is It Salvageable?" *American Journal of Obstetrics & Gynecology* 182, no. 4 (2000): 982–987.

22. Declercq, *Listening to Mothers II*, 31.

23. F. D. Frigoletto and M. F. Greene, "Is There a Sea Change Ahead for Obstetrics and Gynecology?" *Obstetrics & Gynecology* 100, no. 6 (2002): 1342–1343.

24. Lisa H. Schneck, "Strength in Numbers: Medical Group Practices Fill Vital Niche in U.S. Health Care System," MGMA Connex 4, no. 1 (Jan. 2004): 34–43; L. P. Casalino, H. Pham, and G. Bazzoli, "Growth of Single-Specialty Medical Groups," *Health Affairs (Millwood)* 23, no. 2 (2004): 82–90; L. P. Casalino, K. J. Devers, T. K. Lake, M. Reed, and J. J. Stoddard, "Benefits of and Barriers to Large Medical Group Practice in the United States," *Archives of Internal Medicine* 163, no. 16 (2003): 1958–1964.

25. Allison Leibhaber and Joy M. Grossman, *Physicians Moving to Mid-Sized, Single-Specialty Practices, Tracking report no. 18* (Washington, DC: Center for Studying Health System Change, 2007), http://www.hschange.com/CONTENT/941/.

26. R. Finn, "Laborist Movement Poised to Take Off," *Ob/Gyn News* 40, no. 12 (2005): 1; L. Weinstein, "The Laborist: A New Focus of Practice for the Obstetrician," *American Journal of Obstetrics & Gynecology* 188, no. 2 (February 2003): 310–312.

27. E. Hing, D. K. Cherry, and D. A. Woodwell, "National Ambulatory Medical Care Survey: 2004 Summary," *Advance Data* 374 (June 23, 2006): 1–33.

28. Declercq et al., *Listening to Mothers II*, 28.

29. Ibid., 32.

30. Ibid., 56–57.

31. A. Rokade, "Has the Internet Overtaken Other Traditional Sources of Health Information? Questionnaire Survey of Patients Attending ENT Outpatient Clinics," *Clinical Otolaryngology & Allied Sciences* 27, no. 6 (2002): 526–528.

32. Elizabeth Murray, B. Lo, L. Pollack, K. Donelan, J. Catania, M. White et al., "The Impact of Health Information on the Internet on the Physician-Patient Relationship: Patient Perceptions," *Archives of Internal Medicine* 163, no. 14 (July 28, 2003)): 1727–1734.

33. Wertz and Wertz, *Lying-in*, 150–154.

34. Martin Kaufman, *Homeopathy in America: The Rise and Fall of a Medical Heresy* (Baltimore: Johns Hopkins University Press, 1971).

35. Eugene Declercq, "The Trials of Hanna Porn: The Campaign to Abolish Midwifery in Massachusetts" *American Journal of Public Health* 84, no. 6 (June 1994): 1022–1028.

36. Eugene Declercq, Raymond DeVries, Kirsi Viisainen, Helga B. Salvesen, and Sirpa Wrede. "Where to Give Birth? Politics and the Place of Birth," in DeVries et al., eds., *Birth by Design*, 7–27.

37. Boston Women's Health Book Collective, *Our Bodies, Ourselves* (New York: Simon and Schuster, 1973).

38. Irwin Chabon, *Awake and Aware: Participating in Childbirth through Psychoprophylaxis* (New York: Dell, 1972).

39. Grantly Dick-Read, *Childbirth Without Fear: The Principles and Practice of Natural Childbirth* (New York: Harper & Brothers, 1949).

40. Marjorie Karmel, *Thank You, Dr. Lamaze: A Mother's Experiences in Painless Childbirth* (Philadelphia: J. B. Lippincott, 1959).

41. Francine H. Nichols and Sharron Smith Humenick, *Childbirth Education: Practice, Research and Theory*, 2nd ed. (Philadelphia: Saunders; 2000).

42. Eugene R. Declercq, "The Politics of Co-Optation: Strategies for Childbirth Educators," *Birth* 10, no.3 (1983):167–172.

43. Declercq et al., *Listening to Mothers II*, 23–24.

44. Deborah Fallows, "How Women and Men Use the Internet," December 28, 2005, http://www.pewinternet.org/Reports/2005/How-Women-and-Men-Use-the-Internet.aspx.

45. Mary Madden, and Susannah Fox, "Finding Answers Online in Sickness and in Health," May 2, 2006, http://www.pewinternet.org/Reports/2006/Finding-Answers-Online-in-Sickness-and-in-Health.aspx.

46. Mollyann Brodie, Rebecca Flournoy, Drew E. Altman, Robert Blendon, John Benson, Marcus Rosenbaum. "Health Information, the Internet, and the Digital Divide," *Health Affairs (Millwood)*, 19, no. 6 (2000): 255–265.

47. Susannah Fox, "Demographics, Degrees of Internet Access, and Health," Chapel Hill, NC; 2006, June 19–20, 2006, http://www.pewinternet.org/Presentations/2006/Demographics-Degrees-of-Internet-Access-and-Health.aspx.

48. Susannah Fox and Gretchen Livingston, "Latinos Online: Hispanics with Lower Levels of Education and English Proficiency Remain Largely Disconnected from the Internet," (Washington, DC: Pew Research Center, 2007), March 14, 2007, http://pewhispanic.org/files/reports/73.pdf.

49. Susannah Fox, "Health Information Online," Washington, D.C.; 2005 May 17, 2005, http://www.pewinternet.org/Reports/2005/Health-Information-Online.aspx.

50. William Godolphin and Angela Towle, *The Use of the Internet by Prenatal Patients for Health Information and Its Consequences* (Vancouver, British Columbia: Division of Health Care Communication, University of British Columbia; 2005).

51. Heidi Murkoff, *What to Expect When You're Expecting*, 1st ed. (New York: Simon & Schuster, 1984).

52. J. Kantor, "Expecting Trouble: The Book They Love to Hate," *New York Times*, September 15, 2005.

53. Declercq et al., *Listening to Mothers II*, 20.

54. Ibid., 56.

55. Fox, "Latinos Online."

56. B. A. Bettes, V. H. Coleman, S. Zinberg, C. Y. Spong, B. Portnoy, E. DeVoto, et al., "Cesarean Delivery on Maternal Request: Obstetrician-Gynecologists' Knowledge, Perception, and Practice Patterns," *Obstetrics & Gynecology* 109, no. 1 (2007): 57–66.

57. Declercq et al., *Listening to Mothers II*, 23–25.

58. Murray et al., "Impact of Health Information," 1730.

59. A. Broom, "Virtually He@lthy: The Impact of Internet Use on Disease Experience and the Doctor-Patient Relationship," *Qualitative Health Research* 15, no. 3 (2005): 327.

60. A. L. O'Boyle, G. D. Davis, B. C. Calhoun,1 "Informed Consent and Birth: Protecting the Pelvic Floor and Ourselves," *American Journal of Obstetrics & Gynecology* 187, no. 4 (2002): 981–983.

Chapter 8. A Profession of IT's Own

Acknowledgments: Funding has been provided by the National Science Foundation's programs in Sociology and in Law and Social Science (Grant SES-0242033), by an Investigator Award from the Robert Wood Johnson Foundation (Grant #047734), and by seed grants from the Wisconsin Alumni Research Foundation and the University of Wisconsin Center for the Demography of Health and Aging.

1. Stephen Barley, "Technology as an Occasion for Structuring: Evidence from Observation of CT Scanners and the Social Order of Radiology Departments," *Administrative Science Quarterly* 31 (1986): 78–108; Stephen Barley, "The Alignment of Technology and Structure through Roles and Networks," *Administrative Science Quarterly* 35 (1990): 61–103.

2. Andrew Abbott, *The System of Professions: An Essay on the Division of Expert Labor* (Chicago: University of Chicago Press, 1988).

3. Mark C. Suchman and Karen S. Schaepe, "Anticipating the Organizational, Professional and Legal Challenges of Emerging Information Technologies in Health Care" (paper presented at the annual meeting of the Law and Society Association in Vancouver, British Columbia, June 1, 2002, and to the annual meeting of the American Sociological Association in Chicago, Illinois, 2002).

4. Portions of this discussion are drawn from the first author's ongoing collaborative work with W. Richard Scott: Mark C. Suchman and W. Richard Scott, "Beyond Pros and Cons: Constructing an Institutional Model of the Professions" (working paper, Department of Sociology, Brown University, 2009).

5. W. Richard Scott, "Lords of the Dance: Professionals as Institutional Agents," *Organization Studies* 29 (2008): 219–238; Suchman and Scott, "Beyond Pros and Cons."

6. Alexander M. Carr-Saunders and P. A. Wilson, *The Professions* (Oxford: Clarendon Press, 1933); T. H. Marshall, "The Recent History of Professionalism in Relation to Social Structure and Social Policy," *Canadian Journal of Economics and Political Science* 5 (1939): 325–340; William J. Goode, "Community within a Community: The Professions," *American Sociological Review* 22 (1957): 194–200; Ernest Greenwood, "The Attributes of a Profession," *Social Work* 2 (1957): 45–55; Harold L. Wilensky, "The Professionalization of Everyone?" *American Journal of Sociology* 70 (1964): 137–158.

7. Some researchers would expand the list of defining attributes to include such characteristics as collegiality, high status, and fiduciary responsibility. But the seven items listed here constitute the core of most definitions, and additions to the list tend to be either derivative or contested.

8. Because professional world views can, in general, be reduced to the intersection of knowledge/facts and ethics/values, some might dispute whether a world view constitutes a separate defining characteristic of professionalism. We list world view separately here to emphasize that for most professions, knowledge and ethics combine to produce a more encompassing and interconnected belief system than one might expect from considering either knowledge or ethics independently of the other.

9. Marshall, "Recent History of Professionalism"; Talcott Parsons, "Professions," in *International Encyclopedia of the Social Sciences*, ed. D. L. Sills (New York: Free Press, 1968), vol. 12; Wilbert E. Moore, "The Criteria of Professionalism" and "Knowledge and Its Responsibilities," in his book, *The Professions: Roles and Rules* (New York: Russell Sage Foundation, 1970), 3–22, 233–243.

10. Eliot Freidson, *Profession of Medicine: A Study of the Sociology of Applied Knowledge* (New York: Dodd, Mead, 1970); Terence J. Johnson, *Professions and Power* (London: Macmillan, 1972); Magali Sarfatti Larson, *The Rise of Professionalism: A Sociological Analysis* (Berkeley: University of California Press, 1977).

11. John W. Meyer and Brian Rowan, "Institutionalized Organizations: Formal Structure as Myth and Ceremony," *American Journal of Sociology* 83 (1977): 340–363; Paul DiMaggio and Walter W. Powell, "Introduction," in *The New Institutionalism in Organizational Analysis*, ed. Walter W. Powell and Paul DiMaggio (Chicago: University of Chicago Press, 1991); W. Richard Scott, *Institutions and Organizations*, 2d ed. (Thousand Oaks, CA: Sage, 2001).

12. James G. March and Johan P. Olsen, "The New Institutionalism: Organizational Factors in Political Life," *American Political Science Review* 78 (1984): 734–749; Peter A. Hall and Rosemary C. R. Taylor, "Political Science and the Three New Institutionalisms," *Political Studies* 44 (1996): 936–957; Kathleen Thelen, "Historical Institutionalism in Comparative Politics," *Annual Review of Political Science* 2 (1999): 369–404.

13. Douglass North, *Institutions, Institutional Change, and Economic Performance* (Cambridge: Cambridge University Press, 1990); Oliver E. Williamson, *Markets and Hierarchies, Analysis and Antitrust Implications: A Study in the Economics of Internal Organization* (New York: Free Press, 1975); Avner Greif, *Institutions and the Path to the Modern Economy* (New York: Cambridge University Press, 2006).

14. See generally, DiMaggio and Powell, "Introduction" and Scott, *Institutions and Organizations*.

15. Scott, *Institutions and Organizations*; Grief, *Institutions*, 30.

16. Anthony Giddens, *The Constitution of Society: Outline of the Theory of Structuration* (Berkeley: University of California Press, 1984); Ronald L. Jepperson, "Institutions, Institutional Effects, and Institutionalism," in Powell and DiMaggio, eds., *New Institutionalism in Organizational Analysis*; Stephen R. Barley and Pamela S. Tolbert, "Institutionalization and Structuration: Studying the Links between Action and Institution," *Organization Studies* 18 (1997): 93–117.

17. Scott, *Institutions and Organizations*.

18. See, for example, Thomas B. Lawrence and Roy Suddaby, "Institutions and Institutional Work," in *Handbook of Organization Studies*, ed. S. R. Clegg et al., 2nd ed. (London: Sage, 2006), 215–254.

19. Royston Greenwood, Roy Suddaby, and C. R. Hinings, "Theorizing Change: The Role of Professional Associations in the Transformation of Institutionalized Fields," *Academy of Management Journal* 45 (2002): 58–80; Scott, "Professionals as Institutional Agents."

20. To this list, one might add the "softer" coercive devices that have become an increasingly familiar aspect of modern health care finance and organization—service denial, utilization review, cost-containment, etc.

21. Carol A. Heimer, "Competing Institutions: Law, Medicine, and Family in Neonatal Intensive Care," *Law and Society Review* 33 (1999): 17–66.

22. Larson, *Rise of Professionalism*; Abbott, *System of Professions*; DiMaggio and Powell, "Introduction."

23. Abbott, *System of Professions*.

24. Elizabeth Popp, "Creating a National Medical Field: The Associated Apothecaries and Surgeon-Apothecaries, the Provincial Medical and Surgical Association, and the First Professional Project" (working paper, Center for Culture, Organization and Politics, University of California, Berkeley, 2001).

25. Abbott, *System of Professions*.

26. Mark C. Suchman, "Managing Legitimacy: Strategic and Institutional Approaches," *Academy of Management Review* 20 (1995): 571–610.

27. Mary Douglas, *How Institutions Think* (London: Routledge and Kegan Paul, 1987), 52.

28. Malcolm Spector and John I. Kitsuse, *Constructing Social Problems* (Menlo Park, CA: Cummings Publishing, 1977); Stephen Hilgartner and Charles L. Bosk, "The Rise and Fall of Social Problems: A Public Arenas Model," *American Journal of Sociology* 94 (1988): 53–78.

29. Abbott, *System of Professions*.

30. Richard L. Abel, "Comparative Sociology of Legal Professions: An Exploratory Essay," *Law and Social Inquiry* 10 (1985): 5–79.

31. Larson, *Rise of Professionalism*; Richard L. Abel, *American Lawyers* (New York: Oxford University Press, 1989).

32. Lauren B. Edelman, "Legal Ambiguity and Symbolic Structures: Organizational Mediation of Civil Rights Law," *American Journal of Sociology* 97 (1992): 1531–1576; Lauren B. Edelman, Steven E. Abraham, and Howard S. Erlanger, "Professional Construction of the Legal Environment: The Inflated Threat of Wrongful Discharge Doctrine," *Law and Society Review* 26 (1992): 47–83; Frank Dobbin, John R. Sutton, John W. Meyer, and W. Richard Scott, "Equal Opportunity Law and the Construction of Internal Labor Markets," *American Journal of Sociology* 99 (1992): 396–427; Frank Dobbin and John R. Sutton, "The Strength of a Weak State: The Rights Revolution and the Rise of Human Resources Management Divisions," *American Journal of Sociology* 104 (1998): 441–476.

33. Terence C. Halliday, "Six Score Years and Ten: Demographic Transitions in the American Legal Profession, 1850–1980," *Law and Society Review* 20 (1986): 53–78.

34. Calvin Morrill, "Institutional Change Through Interstitial Emergence: The Growth of Alternative Dispute Resolution in American Law, 1965–1995" (paper presented at the annual meeting of the Law and Society Association, Aspen, Colorado, 1998).

35. Abbott, *System of Professions*.

36. The numbers here and in the following section are based on original analyses conducted by the authors using data from the Bureau of Labor Statistics, U.S. Department of Labor, Occupational Employment Statistics, www.bls.gov/oes/ (accessed January 10, 2009).

37. Estimating the size of the HIP workforce from BLS data is an imprecise science. The BLS lists a distinct occupational category only for "medical records and health information technicians," and "technician" is a term of art, meaning that this category excludes most higher-level health-information professionals. For the analyses reported here, we construct additional HIP job categories by breaking out employment numbers *within the health care industry* for several general information-work occupations (see notes to table 8.1). An element of caution is in order, however, because unlike the BLS's technician category, these constructed categories presumably sweep in some information-work that involves health care financing and administration, not direct clinical care.

38. See also Brad Ericson, "2008 Salary Survey: Sunlight on Coders' Compensation," *AAPC Coding Edge* (2008): 19, available at: http://www.aapc.com/documents/ OctCE_Salary%20Survey.pdf (accessed February 5, 2009).

39. DiMaggio, "Constructing an Organizational Field"; Tracey L. Adams, "Inter-Professional Conflict and Professionalization: Dentistry and Dental Hygiene in Ontario," *Social Science and Medicine* 58 (2004): 2243–2252.

40. Halliday, "Demographic Transitions."

41. John Freeman and Michael T. Hannan, "Niche Width and the Dynamics of Organizational Populations," *American Journal of Sociology* 88 (1983): 1116–1145.

42. AHIMA, "AHIMA History," http://www.ahima.org/about/history.asp (accessed February 4, 2009); Carolyn E. Lipscomb, "Professional Boundaries and Medical Records Management," *Journal of the Medical Library Association* 91 (2003): 393–396.

43. Information in this paragraph is drawn primarily from the AHIMA Web site, www.ahima.org.

44. AHIMA, "New Member Profile Results Show HIM Careers Expanding," *AHIMA Advantage* 9 (2005), http://library.ahima.org/xpedio/groups/public/documents/ahima/bok1_027426.hcsp?dDocName=bok1_027426.

45. AHIMA, "Why Get Certified?" http://www.ahima.org/certification/ (accessed February 5, 2009).

46. Information in this paragraph is drawn primarily from the HIMSS Web site, www.himss.org.

47. HIMSS Legacy Workgroup, "History of the Healthcare Information and Management Systems Society (Formerly Hospital Management Systems Society)," http://www.himss.org/content/files/HIMSS_HISTORY.pdf (accessed February 5, 2009).

48. HIMSS Legacy Workgroup, "History of the Healthcare Information and Management Systems Society."

49. HIMSS, "About HIMSS," http://www.himss.org/asp/aboutHimssHome.asp (accessed February 5, 2009).

50. HIMSS Legacy Workgroup, "History of the Healthcare Information and Management Systems Society."

51. Information in this paragraph is drawn primarily from the AMIA Web site, www.amia.org.

52. AAMSI was, itself, the product of a 1981 merger of the Society for Computer Medicine (SCM, founded in 1972) and the Society for Advanced Medical Systems (SAMS, founded in 1977).

53. AMIA, "Member Center: AMIA Has a Rich History of Achievement," http://www2.amia.org/mbrcenter/mbrshp/ (accessed February 5, 2009).

54. AMIA executive staff member, Confidential telephone interview with authors. December 20, 2006.

55. Currently, thirteen of its nineteen board members list university affiliations, compared to three of thirteen for AHIMA, and one of seventeen for HIMSS. See AMIA, "AMIA Board of Directors," http://www.amia.org/inside/leadership (accessed February 5, 2009).

56. AMIA, "AMIA Academic Strategic Leadership Council," http://www.amia.org/inside/initiatives/aslc.asp, and "Academic Forum Introduction," http://www.amia.org/content/academic-forum-introduction (both accessed February 5, 2009).

57. Paul C. Tang, "American Medical Informatics Association State of the Association Meeting," www.amia.org/files/stateslides_06.ppt (accessed February 5, 2009).

58. Glenn R. Carroll, "Concentration and Specialization: Dynamics of Niche Width in Populations of Organizations," *American Journal of Sociology* 90 (1985): 1262–1283; Glenn R. Carroll and Anand Swaminathan, "Why the Microbrewery Movement? Organizational Dynamics of Resource Partitioning in the American Brewing Industry after Prohibition," *American Journal of Sociology* 106 (2000): 712–762; Stanislav D. Dobrev, Tai Young Kim, and Michael T. Hannan, "Dynamics of Niche Width and Resource Partitioning," *American Journal of Sociology* 106 (2001): 1299–1337.

59. Information in this paragraph is drawn primarily from the CHIME Web site, www.cio-chime.org. CHIME, "About CHIME: History of CHIME," http://www.cio-chime.org/chime/about/history.asp (accessed February 5, 2009).

60. CHIME, "Join CHIME: Membership Criteria," http://www.cio-chime.org/JoinCHIME/criteria.asp (accessed February 5, 2009).

61. HIMSS Legacy Workgroup, "History of the Healthcare Information and Management Systems Society."

62. Information in this paragraph is drawn primarily from the AMDIS Web site, www.amdis.org.

63. In one recent survey, 75 percent of CMIOs reported that they continue to practice medicine. Violet L. Shaffer, "Evolving Organization Needs and the Role of CMIO: 2007 AMDIS Gartner Survey Findings," http://www.amdis.org/2007%20AMDIS%20Gartner%20Survey.pdf (accessed February 5, 2009).

64. AAPC, "American Academy of Professional Coders: Home," http://www.aapc.com/ (accessed February 5, 2009).

65. Significantly, however, medical coders are only a disadvantaged occupational group *relative* to their fellow health information professionals. According to a recent survey, in 2007 the average annual salary for medical coders varied from $35,000 to $45,000 depending on region—quite close to the average annual salary of $40,700 in the U.S. economy as a whole. Unlike the average U.S. worker, however, professional coders in most regions experienced salary increases of 15–20 percent from 2007 to 2008. See Ericson, "2008 Salary Survey."

66. AAPC, "Medical Coding Certification," http://www.aapc.com/certification/index.aspx (accessed February 5, 2009); Bureau of Labor Statistics, "Occupational Outlook Handbook, 2008–09 Edition: Medical Records and Health Information Technicians," http://www.stats.bls.gov/oco/ocos103.htm (accessed February 5, 2009).

67. Glenn R. Carroll and Michael T. Hannan, *The Demography of Corporations and Industries* (Princeton, NJ: Princeton University Press, 2000).

68. Figure 8.4 could be read as showing at least a slight inverse relationship between the growth rates of AHIMA and AAPC in the period since 1999. This may reflect the abovementioned competition between those two bodies in the market for coder-certification. However, one should not lose sight of the fact that *both* associations experience significant and monotonic growth throughout this period, suggesting that, despite whatever competition may exist, the game is hardly zero-sum.

69. This count includes only conferences based in the United States. HIMSS has recently launched two international annual conferences, one based in Asia and the other in the Middle East.

70. CHIME, "Events and Education: Past CIO Forum Highlights," http://www.cio-chime.org/events/forum/highlights.asp (accessed February 5, 2009).

71. HIMSS Legacy Workgroup, "History of the Healthcare Information and Management Systems Society."

72. To compile journal counts, we searched the National Library of Medicine's electronic catalog for the specification: (health* OR medic* OR clinic* OR hospital*) AND (informat* OR comput* OR data*). Results were then narrowed by hand and supplemented with a small number of additional journals listed at http://www.informatics-review.com/journals/index.html. To preserve our focus on health information management, we excluded eighteen journals that meet our search criteria but that publish exclusively in the fields of genomics, bioinformatics, or computer imaging and monitoring.

73. Carroll and Hannan, *Demography of Corporations*.

74. These lists are currently confined to the "generalist" associations in the HIP field. As of this writing, none of the more narrowly focused HIP associations (AMDIS,

CHIME, and AAPC) either list, approve, or accredit training programs in their respective areas.

75. AHIMA, "Approved Coding Education Programs," http://www.ahima.org/careers/college_search/search.asp (accessed February 5, 2009).

76. AMIA, "Informatics Academic and Training Programs," http://www.amia.org/informatics/acad%2526training/index.asp (accessed February 5, 2009).

77. HIMSS, "Directory of Academic Programs in HIMSS-Related Disciplines," http://www.himss.org/content/files/EducatorsSIGdirectory.pdf (accessed February 5, 2009).

78. CAHIIM, "Directory of Academic Programs," http://www.cahiim.org/directory/ (accessed February 5, 2009).

79. This count is complicated by the fact that several educational institutions offer HIP training opportunities through multiple programs—for example a health information management program in the business school and a nursing informatics program in the school of nursing. In addition, many programs offer multiple types of educational opportunities (including everything from short online courses to research fellowships and post-docs) and award multiple degrees. Our discussion therefore distinguishes between the number of educational institutions, the number of programs, and the number of educational opportunities. In general, however, we focus on the number of programs, because this indicator, we believe, is the most reflective both of student experiences and of the structure of professional knowledge.

80. LCME, "Overview: Accreditation and the LCME," http://www.lcme.org/overview .htm (accessed February 5, 2009).

81. NLNAC, "About NLNAC," http://www.nlnac.org/About%20NLNAC/whatsnew.htm (accessed February 5, 2009); CCNE, "Annual Report," http://www.aacn.nche.edu/Media/pdf/AnnualReport08.pdf (accessed February 5, 2009).

82. Admittedly, an account of expertise may certainly imply that lay regulation will be imperfect; however, imperfect lay regulation may still be preferable to *unethical* professional self-regulation. Thus, even technocratic arguments for professional self-regulation assume some degree of professional ethicality.

83. Simon de Lusignan, Tom Chan, Alice Theadom, and Neil Dhoul, "The Roles of Policy and Professionalism in the Protection of Processed Clinical Data: A Literature Review," *International Journal of Medical Informatics* 76 (2007): 261–268.

84. For example, Hannu Vuori, "Privacy, Confidentiality and Automated Health Information Systems," *Journal of Medical Ethics* 3 (1977): 174–178; Vernon Coleman, "Why Patients Should Keep Their Own Records," *Journal of Medical Ethics* 10 (1984): 27–28.

85. For example, Eike-Henner W. Kluge, "Medical Informatics and Education: The Profession as Gate-Keeper," *Methods of Information in Medicine* 28 (1989): 196–201; Eike-Henner W. Kluge, "Health Information, Privacy, Confidentiality and Ethics," *International Journal of Bio-Medical Computing* 35 (1994): 23–27; Eike-Henner W. Kluge, "Health Information, the Fair Information Principles and Ethics," *Methods of Information in Medicine* 33 (1994): 336–345; Mary Curran and Kent Curran, "The Ethics of Information," *Journal of Nursing Administration* 21 (1994): 47–49; Lawrence O. Gostin, "Health Information Privacy," *Cornell Law Review* 80 (1995): 451–528.

86. Audrey R. Chapman, ed., *Health Care and Information Ethics: Protecting Fundamental Human Rights* (Kansas City, MO: Sheen and Ward, 1997).

87. Laurinda B. Harman, ed., *Ethical Challenges in the Management of Health Information* (Gaithersburg, MD: Aspen Publishers, 2001).

88. Eike-Henner W. Kluge, "Fostering a Security Culture: A Model Code of Ethics for Health Information Professionals," *International Journal of Medical Informatics* 49 (1998): 105–110; Eike-Henner W. Kluge, "Professional Codes for Electronic HC Record Protection: Ethical, Legal, Economic and Structural Issues," *International Journal of Medical Informatics* 60 (2000): 85–96; Eike-Henner W. Kluge, *The Ethics of Electronic Patient Records* (New York: Peter Lang, 2001); Eike-Henner W. Kluge, *A Handbook of Ethics for Health Informatics Professionals* (Bristol: British Computer Society Health Informatics Committee, 2003).

89. Kazimierz Trzęsicki, "Medical Informatics Ethics and Its Subject," *Annales Academiae Medicae Bialostocensis* 50 (2005): 20–22.

90. AHIMA, "Code of Ethics," http://library.ahima.org/xpedio/groups/public/documents/ahima/bok1_024277.hcsp?dDocName=bok1_024277 (accessed February 5, 2009); IMIA, "The IMIA Code of Ethics for Health Information Professionals," http://www.imia.org/pubdocs/Ethics_Eng.pdf (accessed February 5, 2009).

91. AMIA, "AMIA Code of Ethics," http://www.amia.org/inside/code (accessed February 5, 2009).

92. HIMSS, "HIMSS Code of Ethics," www2.himss.org/private/chapters/download/bylaws/appendixB.doc (accessed February 5, 2009).

93. AAPC, "Medical Coding Code of Ethics," http://www.aapc.com/aboutus/code-of-ethics.aspx (accessed February 6, 2009). Other associations in the field have also promulgated short ethical codes, similar to the AAPC's 250-word offering. For example, the Association of Health Information Outsourcing Services (AHIOS) has a 390-word code, www.ahios.org/about/code-ethics-standards.php, and the Society for Clinical Data Management (SCDM) has a 250-word statement of commitments, http://www.scdm.org/about/.

94. IMIA, "IMIA Code of Ethics," preamble, section 3.

95. AHIMA, "Code of Ethics," preamble, paragraph 1.

96. AHIMA, "Code of Ethics," Principle 3.

97. IMIA, "IMIA Code of Ethics," Part I B 2–4.

98. IMIA, "IMIA Code of Ethics," Part II A 9.

99. IMIA, "IMIA Code of Ethics," Part II B 1–5.

100. AHIMA, "Code of Ethics," Principle 5.3.

101. AHIMA, "Code of Ethics," Principle 5.1.

102. AHIMA, "Code of Ethics," Principle 1.2.

103. AHIMA, "Code of Ethics," Principle 4.6.

104. See generally each organization's Web site on credentials: AHIMA, "Why Get Certified?" http://www.ahima.org/certification/ (accessed February 7, 2009); and AAPC, "Medical Coding Certification" http://www.aapc.com/certification/index.aspx (accessed February 7, 2009).

105. HIMSS, "CPHIMS Certification," http://www.himss.org/ASP/certification_cphims.asp (accessed February 6, 2009). Other associations in the field offer additional specialized credentials, such as the Society of Clinical Data Management's "Certified Clinical Data Manager" (CCDM) designation, and the large array of coding certifications in various medical specialty areas from the Board of Medical Specialty Coding (BMSC), the Professional Association of Healthcare Coding Specialists (PAHCS), and the National Cancer Registrar's Association (NCRA). See BLS, "Medical Records and Health Information Technicians." While it may be noteworthy that several of the "high end" HIP associations—AMDIS, AMIA, and CHIME—do *not* operate credential programs, this fact is not particularly surprising in light of more potent

non-HIP credentials (such as M.D.s, Ph.D.s, and MBAs) held by many of these associations' members.

106. Credential requirements for AAPC, AHIMA, and HIMSS can be found, respectively, at: AAPC, "Medical Coding Certification"; AHIMA, "Why Get Certified?"; and HIMSS, "CPHIMS Certification: Become Certified," http://www.himss.org/ASP/certification_cphimsApply.asp (accessed February 6, 2009).

107. CAHIIM, "CAHIIM Standards," http://www.cahiim.org/standards/ (accessed February 6, 2009).

108. AHIMA, "Curriculum Model: Baccalaureate Degree Education in Health Information Management," http://www.cahiim.org/resources/documents/HITBacc ModelCurriculum.pdf (accessed February 6, 2009); AHIMA, "Curriculum Model: Associate Degree Education in Health Information Management," http://www.cahiim .org/resources/documents/HITAssocModelCurriculum.pdf (accessed February 6, 2009); AHIMA, "HIM Baccalaureate Degree Knowledge Cluster Content and Competency Levels," http://library.ahima.org/xpedio/groups/public/documents/ ahima/bok1_025411.doc. (accessed February 6, 2009).

109. Ericson, "2008 Salary Survey," 19.

110. Paul Wing, Margie Langelier, Tracey Continelli, and David Armstrong, "Data for Decisions: The HIM Workforce and Workplace: Summary of the Responses to the 2002 AHIMA Member Survey," http://library.ahima.org/xpedio/groups/public/ documents/ahima/bok1_018947.pdf (accessed February 6, 2009).

111. Wing et al., "2002 AHIMA Member Survey." Membership surveys, of course, must be read with caution, because individuals who belong to professional associations and participate in professional self-portraits may not represent a fair cross-section of the field as a whole. Presumably, the role of credentialing in other HIP worksites is somewhat lower than in the sites described by AAPC and AHIMA members.

112. Department of Health and Human Services, Office of Inspector General, "OIG Draft Supplemental Compliance Program Guidance for Hospitals," 69 Fed. Reg. 32012–32031 at 32030 (2004).

113. Hawaii Revised Statutes § 431:9–243 (2008).

114. CCHIT, "About CCHIT," http://www.cchit.org/about/index.asp (accessed February 6, 2009).

115. Carroll and Hannan, *Demography of Corporations*; Suchman, "Managing Legitimacy."

116. D. J. Hickson, C. R. Hinings, C. A. Lee, R. E. Schneck, and J. M. Pennings, "A Strategic Contingencies Theory of Intraorganizational Power," *Administrative Science Quarterly* 16 (1971): 216–229.

117. Edelman et al., "Professional Construction of the Legal Environment."

118. Elisabeth S. Clemens and James M. Cook, "Politics and Institutionalism: Explaining Durability and Change," *Annual Review of Sociology* 25 (1999): 441–466; Scott, *Institutions and Organizations*, 181–204; Greenwood et al., "Theorizing Change."

119. W. Richard Scott, "Reactions to Supervision in a Heteronomous Professional Organization," *Administrative Science Quarterly* 10 (1965): 65–81.

120. The authors wish to thank Karen Schaepe for conducting much of the fieldwork that contributed to this section.

About the Contributors

David Blumenthal, director of the Institute for Health Policy at Massachusetts General Hospital/Partners HealthCare System, is professor of health care policy and the Samuel O. Thier Professor of Medicine at Harvard Medical School. He is also director of the Harvard University Interfaculty Program for Health Systems Improvement. A member of the Institute of Medicine, Dr. Blumenthal serves on several editorial boards, including the *American Journal of Medicine* and *Journal of Health Politics, Policy, and Law.* He is also a national correspondent for the *New England Journal of Medicine.* He was a senior advisor to the Obama campaign in health policy. His research interests include the dissemination of health information technology, quality management in health care, the determinants of physician behavior, access to health services, and the extent and consequences of academic-industrial relationships in the health sciences.

Eugene Declercq is professor and assistant dean for doctoral education at the Boston University School of Public Health. He also serves on the faculty of obstetrics and gynecology at the Boston University School of Medicine. He was awarded a Robert Wood Johnson Investigator Award in Health Policy Research to study policy and practice related to cesarean section in the United States and has served as lead author of two national studies of women's experiences in childbirth titled *Listening to Mothers.*

Matthew Dimick is a Ph.D. candidate in sociology at the University of Wisconsin–Madison. His substantive interests are in comparative political economy, work and occupations, and the economic and sociological analysis of law and legal institutions; his methodological interests lie primarily in game theory and comparative-historical analysis. He is currently completing a dissertation on the relationship between labor law and labor-union democracy in the United States and Great Britain.

Mark Hall is the Fred D. and Elizabeth L. Turnage Professor of Law and Public Health at Wake Forest University, where he has appointments in the Schools of Law, Medicine, and Management. Professor Hall specializes in health care law and public policy, with a focus on economic, regulatory and organizational issues. He is the lead editor of the original textbook in the field, *Health Care Law and Ethics,* and he has written books on various aspects of health care law and public policy. He is currently studying the legal and ethical implications of consumer-driven health care under a Robert Wood Johnson Foundation Investigator Award in Health Policy Research.

Kristin Madison is a professor at the University of Pennsylvania Law School and a senior fellow at the Leonard Davis Institute of Health Economics. Her primary areas of interest include the structure of health care organizations, the dissemination of health-related information, and the evolution of health care regulation. Her current research focuses on legal and policy issues related to health care quality reporting.

Michael W. Painter, a physician, attorney and health care policy advocate, is a senior program officer and a senior member of the RWJF Quality/Equality Team. In 2003–2004, Painter was a Robert Wood Johnson Foundation Health Policy Fellow with the office of Senator William H. Frist, M.D., former majority leader. Prior to that, he was the chief of medical staff at the Seattle Indian Health Board, a community health center serving urban American Indians and Alaska Natives. He has a clinical faculty appointment with the University of Washington, Department of Family Medicine. Painter earned a J.D. from Stanford Law School and an M.D. from the University of Washington. He received his residency training at the Providence Family Medicine Residency in Seattle, and is a board-certified family physician. He earned a B.A. in economics and mathematics from Vanderbilt University, graduating summa cum laude, and is a member of Phi Beta Kappa.

Marc A. Rodwin is a professor of law at Suffolk University Law School in Boston. He is the author of *Conflicts of Interest and the Future of Medicine: The United States, France, and Japan* (2010) and *Medicine, Money and Morals: Physicians' Conflicts of Interest* (1993) and has published articles on the relation between law, ethics, and markets. His research is on health care consumer voice and representation; the pharmaceutical industry; accountability in managed care; consumer protection in health care; medical malpractice; and ownership of patient health data.

Rodwin has testified before Congress and served on government commissions and advisory boards including the Food and Drug Administration and the Indiana Commission on Hospital Antitrust. He has participated in meetings of the National Academy of Science–Institute of Medicine, the American Bar Association, the Agency for Health Care Policy and Research, the American College of Physicians, and the Health Care Financial Management Association. He holds a Ph.D. from Brandeis University, a J.D. from the University of Virginia Law School, a B.A., M.A. from Oxford University, and a B.A. from Brown University.

Sara Rosenbaum is the Harold and Jane Hirsh Professor and founding chair of the Department of Health Policy, George Washington University School of Public Health and Health Services. Professor Rosenbaum has devoted her career to issues of health law and policy affecting low income, minority, and medically underserved populations. Between 1993 and 1994, Professor Rosenbaum worked for President Clinton, directing the legislative drafting of the Health Security Act and developing the Vaccines for Children program. She also served on the Presidential Transition Team for President-Elect Obama. In 2009 she was named one of the founding Commissioners of the Medicaid and CHIP Payment and

Access Commission, which advises Congress on federal Medicaid and CHIP policy. She has authored numerous articles and books, among them, *Law and the American Health Care System* (Foundation Press, New York), a widely used health law textbook.

David J. Rothman is the president of the Institute on Medicine as a Profession (IMAP), Bernard Schoenberg Professor of Social Medicine at Columbia College of Physicians & Surgeons, and a professor of history at Columbia University. Trained in American Social History at Harvard University, Rothman first explored the history of mental hospitals, prisons, and almshouses (*The Discovery of the Asylum* (1971), *Conscience and Convenience* (1980), and *The Willowbrook Wars* [1984, co-authored with Sheila M. Rothman]).

Rothman joined the medical school faculty in 1983 and his subsequent work has examined the history of health care practices and health policy. He has published *Strangers at the Bedside* (1991); *Beginnings Count* (1997), and *The Pursuit of Perfection* (2003, co-authored with Sheila Rothman). David Rothman's other scholarly and policy interests include the history and ethics of human experimentation, as well as issues of human rights in medicine. Together with Sheila Rothman, he co-authored *Trust Is Not Enough* (2006).

Rothman is now addressing the role of professionalism in medicine. With an endowment from the Open Society Institute and George Soros, IMAP is dedicated to making professionalism a field and a force. His publications in this area include: "Medical Professionalism; Focusing on the Real Issues" (2000); "New Federal Guidelines for Physician-Pharmaceutical Industry Relations" (2005, coauthored with Susan Chimonas); "Marketing HPV Vaccine: Implications for Adolescent Health and Medical Professionalism" (coauthored with Sheila Rothman, 2009). He co-authored "Health Industry Practices that Create Conflicts of Interest: A Policy Proposal for Academic Medical Centers" (2006) and "Professional Medical Associations and Their Relationships with Industry: A Proposal for Controlling Conflicts of Interest" (2009).

Sheila M. Rothman is a professor of sociomedical sciences at the Joseph L. Mailman School of Public Health at Columbia University. Her research interests include human rights (*Trust Is Not Enough: Bringing Human Rights to Medicine*, 2006), organ transplantation (*The Hidden Costs of Organ Sales*, 2006), and most recently the relationships between consumer health organizations and the pharmaceutical industry.

Natassia M. Rozario is currently a fellow with the American India Foundation, where she is working with the NGO Saath to improve access to primary health care among slum communities of Ahmedabad, India. She previously worked with Drs. David and Sheila Rothman on the topics of living organ donation and conflicts of interest between the medical field and the pharmaceutical industry. Rozario graduated from Columbia with a B.A. in political science and has an M.P.H. from the Johns Hopkins University.

Mark C. Suchman is professor of sociology at Brown University, where he is a member of the core faculty in Commerce, Organizations, and Entrepreneurship and organizer of the Brown Legal Studies Seminar. From 1999 to 2001, he was a Robert Wood Johnson Foundation Scholar in Health Policy Research at Yale University. His research interests center on the relationship between law and organizations, particularly the role of legal institutions in formally and informally legitimating innovation and entrepreneurship in the information technology, nanotechnology, and health care sectors. He is currently engaged in a multi-year project on the organizational, professional, and legal challenges of new information technologies in health care, with a particular focus on hospital responses to HIPAA. He has also written on the role of lawyers in Silicon Valley, on litigation ethics, and on the "internalization" of law within corporate bureaucracies.

Nancy Tomes is professor and chair of the history department at the State University of New York at Stony Brook. She is the author of *A Generous Confidence: Thomas Story Kirkbride and the Art of Asylum Keeping* (1984), *Madness in America: Cultural and Medical Perceptions of Mental Illness before 1914*, co-authored with Lynn Gamwell (1995), and *The Gospel of Germs: Men, Women, and the Microbe in American Life* (1998). She is currently finishing a book on the rise of the twentieth-century health consumer.

Index

Breinigsville, PA USA
05 August 2010
243015BV00002B/2/P